Person-Centred Dementia Care

Bradford Dementia Group Good Practice Guides

Under the editorship of Murna Downs, Chair in Dementia Studies at the University of Bradford, this series constitutes a set of accessible, jargon-free, evidence-based good practice guides for all those involved in the care of people with dementia and their families. The series draws together a range of evidence including the experience of people with dementia and their families, practice wisdom, and research and scholarship to promote quality of life and quality of care.

Bradford Dementia Group offer undergraduate and post graduate degrees in dementia studies and short courses in person-centred care and Dementia Care Mapping, alongside study days in contemporary topics. Information about these can be found on www.bradford.ac.uk/acad/health/dementia.

other titles in the series

Design for Nature in Dementia Care
Garuth Chalfont
ISBN 978 1 84310 571 8

The Pool Activity Level (PAL) Instrument for Occupational Profiling
A Practical Resource for Carers of People with Cognitive Impairment
3rd edition
Jackie Pool
ISBN 978 1 84310 594 7

Involving Families in Care Homes
A Relationship-Centred Approach to Dementia Care
Bob Woods, John Keady and Diane Seddon
ISBN 978 1 84310 229 8

Ethical Issues in Dementia Care
Making Difficult Decisions
Julian C. Hughes and Clive Baldwin
ISBN 978 1 84310 357 8

Healing Arts Therapies and Person-Centred Dementia Care
Edited by Anthea Innes and Karen Hatfield
ISBN 978 1 84310 038 6

Primary Care and Dementia
Steve Iliffe and Vari Drennan
Foreword by Murna Downs
ISBN 978 1 85302 997 4

of related interest

Understanding Learning Disability and Dementia
Developing Effective Interventions
Diana Kerr
ISBN 978 1 84310 442 1

The Simplicity of Dementia
A Guide for Family and Carers
Huub Buijssen
ISBN 978 1 84310 321 9

Person-Centred Dementia Care

Making Services Better

Dawn Brooker

Jessica Kingsley Publishers
London and Philadelphia

First published in 2007
by Jessica Kingsley Publishers
116 Pentonville Road
London N1 9JB, UK
and
400 Market Street, Suite 400
Philadelphia, PA 19106, USA

www.jkp.com

Library of Congress Cataloging in Publication Data

Brooker, Dawn, 1959-
 Person-centred dementia care : making services better / Dawn Brooker.
  p. ; cm.
 Includes bibliographical references and index.
 ISBN-13: 978-1-84310-337-0 (alk. paper)
 ISBN-10: 1-84310-337-0 (alk. paper)
 1. Dementia--Treatment. 2. Dementia--Patients--Care. 3. Dementia--Nursing. I. Title.
 [DNLM: 1. Dementia--nursing. 2. Nurse-Patient Relations. 3. Nursing Care--methods. 4.
Patient-Centered Care--methods. WM 220 B872p 2007]
 RC521.B7644 2007
 616.8'3--dc22

                                                                    2006034310

British Library Cataloguing in Publication Data
A CIP catalogue record for this book is available from the British Library

ISBN 978 1 84310 337 0

Printed and bound in Great Britain by
MPG Books Limited, Cornwall

Contents

Acknowledgements

This book has been in my mind for years. It has been shaped by many discussions with many people – family members, clients and by my colleagues in the field of dementia care. The groundwork came from my time in Birmingham working as a clinical psychologist within a multi-disciplinary team who, looking back, appear now to have been quite ahead of their time – Hilary Nissenbaum, Carole Dinshaw, Jan Oyebode, Claire Crawley and Paul Pyke to name just a few. Over the years those clinical psychologists working with older people – particularly Bob Woods, Linda Clare, Esme Moniz-Cook, Mike Bender, Rik Cheston, Graham Stokes, Polly Kaiser, Nicky Bradbury and Ian James – have provided a bed-rock for developing these ideas.

The person who helped me make most sense of the challenging terrain, first through his writing and later through his mentorship, was undoubtedly the late Tom Kitwood. Without Tom, this book simply would not have existed. Tom gave me a map which led eventually to many years of work with the Bradford Dementia Group. Murna Downs ensured the book was written, and her editing and wise counsel have been invaluable. My other colleagues and friends at Bradford have supplied many thoughts and ideas along the way, and have graciously supplied me with the space to write – Claire Surr, Paul Edwards, Caroline Baker, Hazel May and Jean Martin have been my constant companions in the writing. Errollyn Bruce and Ruth Bartlett provided some much needed inspiration too. Christine Bryden's writing was both an inspiration and a validation. Thanks especially to Caroline Baker for making the connections between Christine's writing and our thoughts on positive person work. The wider community of Dementia Care Mapping (DCM) trainers and practitioners – Lisa Heller, Jane Fossey, Tracy Packer, Elizabeth Barnett, Tessa Perrin, Tracey Lintern, Eva Bonde-Nielsen,

Yutaka Mizuno, Christian Muller-Hergl, Roseann Kasayka and Virginia Moore have shaped my thinking in ways that are too many to count.

All the many people and care providers who generously provided feedback on the early stages of the VIPS tool are the ones to thank if the tool proves to be of use in practice. My work with practitioners at the ExtraCare Charitable Trust, and lately with a very committed group at the Commission for Social Care Inspection, has undoubtedly sharpened my thinking and, I hope, made the output more practicable.

Finally, thanks to my lovely husband and son and to my mum for understanding my compulsion to write this all down.

Part 1

Unpacking What We Mean by Person-Centered Care

1

What is Person-Centred Care?

Person-centred care is written into policy documents, training courses, mission statements, care-planning tools, job descriptions and protocols in almost every part of the UK care scene. This is particularly true for services for people living with dementia. It seems that any dementia care initiative has to claim to be 'pc' (person-centred) in order to be 'PC' (politically correct). Many of us live with the uneasy knowledge, however, that, although the words sound good, the lived experience of care for people with dementia – particularly for those living in long-term care – is anything but person-centred.

The essential elements of person-centred care: VIPS

As with many terms that are frequently used, there is a tendency for person-centred care to mean different things to different people in different contexts. In my discussions with practitioners, researchers, people with dementia and their families, it is obvious that the concepts in person-centred care are not easy to understand or articulate in a straightforward manner. To some, it means individualised care; to others, it is a value base. There are people who see it as a set of techniques to use with people with dementia, and to others it is a phenomenological perspective and a means of communication.

The definition of person-centred care is not a straightforward one. Person-centred care as it relates to people with dementia has become a composite term and any definition needs to take this into consideration. The elements of the composite can become so long-winded, however, that the definition loses focus and shape.

A couple of years ago, I was asked to write a review on person-centred care. What struck me very quickly in my reading was that there was no one accepted definition of what this much used term meant. In looking at a large number of authors who were writing about person-centred care, it appeared to me that a contemporary definition of person-centred dementia care describes four essential elements (Brooker 2004):

1. Valuing people with dementia and those who care for them; promoting their citizenship rights and entitlements regardless of age or cognitive impairment.

2. Treating people as individuals; appreciating that all people with dementia have a unique history and personality, physical and mental health, and social and economic resources, and that these will affect their response to neurological impairment.

3. Looking at the world from the perspective of the person with dementia; recognising that each person's experience has its own psychological validity, that people with dementia act from this perspective, and that empathy with this perspective has its own therapeutic potential.

4. Recognising that all human life, including that of people with dementia, is grounded in relationships, and that people with dementia need an enriched social environment which both compensates for their impairment and fosters opportunities for personal growth.

Person-centred care encompasses four major elements, all of which have been defined as person-centred care in and of themselves by some writers. These elements are:

V A value base that asserts the absolute value of all human lives regardless of age or cognitive ability.

I An individualised approach, recognising uniqueness.

P Understanding the world from the perspective of the service user.

S Providing a social environment that supports psychological needs.

I have called the four parts, 'elements of person-centred care'. This is in recognition of the fact that all these things can and do exist independently of each other. When they are brought together, however, they define the powerful culture of a person-centred approach to care. Continuing the style that Professor Tom Kitwood had for representing complex ideas in the form of equations, this can also be expressed as

$$PCC \text{ (person-centred care)} = V + I + P + S$$

This equation does not give a pre-eminence of any element over another – they are all contributory. Of course, the acronym VIPS also stands for Very Important Persons which is an easier way of defining the outcome of person-centred care for people with dementia.

In this opening chapter, I look at the origins of person-centred care and the proliferation of care processes and tools that now fall under this heading. The rest of the book is concerned with spelling out what the four elements of person-centred care look like in practice. It is only by being crystal clear about what we mean by person-centred care that we can tell whether the reality lives up to the rhetoric.

The origins of person-centred care

Person-centred care has its origins in the work of Carl Rogers (Rogers 1961) and client-centred counselling. It was the late Professor Tom Kitwood, the founder of the Bradford Dementia Group, who first used the term 'person-centred' in relation to people with dementia. Writing in the year before his death, Kitwood (1997a) said that he used the term 'person-centred' in the context of dementia care to bring together ideas and ways of working with the lived experience of people with dementia that emphasised communication and relationships. The term was intended to be a direct reference to Rogerian psychotherapy with its emphasis on authentic contact and communication.

Kitwood's work was part of the groundswell of psychosocial approaches to dementia care that came into being during the 1980s and 1990s. Reality Orientation (Holden and Woods 1988) was, in part, a response to offer reassurance to the person with dementia, and a means of decreasing disorientation. Validation therapy (Feil 1993) and resolution therapy (Stokes and Goudie 1990) emphasised the importance of using the experience of the person with dementia as the starting point. Work on individualised care planning and social role valorisation, with its roots in the learning disabilities field, quickly caught on with those working in services for older people who were concerned to understand the people they cared for at a deeper level, and to provide them with opportunities for leading a valued life.

The disability rights movement and the growing dissatisfaction with institutionalised care led to various codes of practice from the Kings Fund in the UK during the 1980s that emphasised the rights of people with dementia to live well. The work of Steven Sabat (Sabat 1994) was influential in shaping thinking about the impact of social environments on people with dementia. As far back as 1985, Joanne Rader and colleagues (Rader, Doan and Schwab 1985) used the term 'agenda behaviour' to highlight the goal-seeking driving much of the behaviour of people with dementia. The 'Pioneer Network' in the USA has been working on changing the culture of nursing-home care for many years (http://pioneernetwork.net). The ideas of Bill Thomas and the Eden Alternative (Thomas 1996) give the experience of the person with dementia a centrality that was absent from approaches that had seen dementia care as a set of problems to be managed.

The ideas that underpin person-centred approaches to care have been with us for a while. It is easy to forget how radical these ideas were when they were first described. Person-centred care was part of a wider movement during the last decades of the 20th century that recognised that people with dementia could benefit from psychological approaches, that they had human rights and that they proposed a challenge to dehumanising care practice which had not been seen previously. Person-centred care has come to encompass all these elements in a short-hand phrase for what is now considered to be good quality care for people with dementia.

Themes from Kitwood

Tom Kitwood provided a theoretical underpinning to the practice of person-centred dementia care. He published a continuous stream of articles in prominent journals during the 1980s and 90s (Kitwood 1987a; 1987b; 1988; 1989; 1990a; 1990b; 1993a; 1993b; 1993c; 1995a; 1995b). He brought these ideas together in his most well-known book, *Dementia Reconsidered: The Person Comes First* (1997a).

om Kitwood was undoubtedly a major influence in developing the cornerstones on which person-centred care now sits: the importance of maintaining personhood; the Enriched Model of dementia; the recognition of the power of Malignant Social Psychology; striving to take the stand-point of the person with dementia, and the description of New Culture care, were a way of articulating the theoretical argument for person-centred approaches that had not been done before. These are now briefly reviewed.

Personhood

Kitwood was also the first writer to use the term 'personhood' in relation to people with dementia. He defined personhood as, 'A standing or status that is bestowed upon one human being, by others, in the context of relationship and social being. It implies recognition, respect and trust' (Kitwood 1997a, p.8).

The primary outcome of person-centred care for people with dementia is to maintain their personhood in the face of declining mental powers. There is an assumption in person-centred care that people with dementia have the capacity to experience relative well-being and ill-being. A simplistic biological model would interpret the expression of ill-being as a random occurrence or as a sign of brain pathology. In person-centred care, the assumption is made that behaviour has meaning. According to Kitwood, high levels of challenging behaviour, distress or apathy occur more commonly in care settings that are not supportive of personhood. In care environments that are supportive of personhood, we expect to see a greater preponderance of well-being and social confidence. This theme is picked up in Chapter 2 when I consider how people with dementia are valued by society generally, and how care providers need to make the valuing of the quality of lives of people with dementia their explicit business if they are serious about providing person-centred care.

The Enriched Model of dementia

Tom Kitwood described the Enriched Model of dementia. This challenged the prevailing assumption in the 1980s that dementia could be understood simply by the degree of loss of brain cortex, what Kitwood called 'the standard paradigm'. The Enriched Model recognised the multiplicity of factors which affect a person's experience of dementia including neurological impairment, physical health, the individual's biography and personality, and the social environment in which they live. At the time when Kitwood first wrote about the Enriched Model, it was thought that little could be done to arrest neurological impairment. The Enriched Model provided the opportunity to maximise well-being by focusing on the other dimensions that affect a person's quality of life. The person-centred approach sees dementia as a condition that needs to be understood from a biological, a psychological and a sociological (bio-psychosocial) perspective, and to recognise that all these perspectives interact to determine the person's experience of the condition. This theme of the uniqueness of experience is discussed in Chapter 3 when I look at the necessity of providing individualised care for those receiving services if their needs are to be supported in a way that is person-centred.

Malignant Social Psychology (MSP)

Personhood is undermined when individual needs and rights are not considered, when powerful negative emotions are ignored or invalidated, and when increasing isolation from human relationships occurs. Kitwood described the various common ways that he had observed personhood being undermined in care settings, coining the phrase 'Malignant Social Psychology' as an umbrella term. MSP includes episodes where people are intimidated, outpaced, not responded to, infantilised, labelled, disparaged, blamed, manipulated, invalidated, disempowered, overpowered, disrupted, objectified, stigmatised, ignored, banished and mocked.

Very few people would wish to deliberately subject other people to MSP. Despite this, in the care of people with dementia around the world, it occurs with surprising regularity. The MSP list is a depressingly familiar one to people working in care. Many care practitioners have a heart-sink feeling when they first read this list. This is due to the realisation that most of us who have worked in dementia care for a number of years have been guilty of most of these things at some point or another.

Kitwood was at pains to say that episodes of MSP are very rarely done with any malicious intent. Rather, episodes of MSP become interwoven into the care culture. This way of responding to people with dementia gets learnt in the same way that new staff learn to fold sheets. If you are a new staff member in a nursing home, you learn how to communicate with people with dementia from other staff with whom you work. If their communication style with residents is one that is characterised by infantilisation and outpacing, then you will follow their lead. The malignancy in MSP is that it eats away at the personhood of those being cared for, and also that it spreads from one member of staff to another very quickly.

The root of MSP lies within our societal values. People with dementia are not valued in a society where youth and intellectual prowess receive the highest accolades. At best, people with dementia are ignored by society. At worst, they are discriminated against. This is society's response to people with dementia generally, and it has all too often become the professional caring response. In care settings, this lack of value manifests itself as MSP.

Frequent episodes of MSP undermine personhood, decrease well-being and increase ill-being. Kitwood postulated that the increasing isolation that resulted from MSP could in itself lead to a loss of function. At its worst, it leads to a radical depersonalisation of people with dementia, and reconfirms to wider society its belief that these people are less than human.

dementia needs to be heard directly in shaping and developing services has become an accepted way of working, if not always easy to achieve in practice (Mozley *et al.* 1999).

More and more direct accounts of what it is like to live with dementia are beginning to appear. One of the richest accounts comes from the Australian writer, Christine Bryden, in her book *Dancing with Dementia* (2005). Christine was formerly a top civil servant who was diagnosed with dementia at the age of 46. Ten years later, Christine describes her journey with dementia as a dance, whereby both she and her husband Paul have had to change their steps along the way to form the pattern of the dance. To help illustrate some of the key issues in person-centred care, quotes from Dancing with Dementia are included thoughout this book.

> Each person with dementia is travelling a journey deep into the core of their spirit, away from the complex cognitive outer layer that once defined them, through the jumble and tangle of emotions created through their life experiences, into the centre of their being, into what truly gives them meaning in life. Many of us seek earnestly for this sense of the present time, the sense of 'now', of how to live each moment and treasure it as if it were the only experience to look at and to wonder at. But this is the experience of dementia, life in the present without a past or future. (Bryden 2005, p.11)

Dementia Care Mapping (DCM)

Bradford Dementia Group in the UK has continued to provide training in DCM and supporting and developing its use in practice to support person-centred care. Training is also available in the USA, Germany, Australia, Denmark, Switzerland and Japan. People from many other countries have taken DCM courses including Finland, Norway, Sweden, Austria, Spain, Portugal, Ireland, Luxembourg, Holland, Belgium, Italy, Canada, New Zealand, China, Singapore, Taiwan and South Korea. Anthea Innes provides a useful cross-cultural perspective on DCM (Innes 2003). The published evidence base concerning the use of DCM continues to grow (Brooker 2005). In recent years, DCM has been revised and updated. This updating was based on current best practice, the research literature, international working groups and thorough field testing of the revised method and training (Brooker and Surr 2006). The revised method places much more emphasis on the ways care workers can uphold personhood and ensure that DCM is an inclusive process.

Therapeutic approach

There is an increasing number of structured or therapeutic activity-based interventions that have been utilised with people with dementia, with the aim of promoting person-centred care. Reminiscence has been a popular approach (Woods *et al.* 2005). Creative activities that employ one or a combination of media such as music (Aldridge 2000; Sherratt, Thornton and Hatton 2004a and 2004b), art, writing (Allan and Killick 2000) dance and movement (Coaten 2001) or drama (Batson 1998), which can be combined with reminiscence (Chaudhury 2003; Coaten 2001) have also proliferated. Cognitive stimulation therapy, which aims to be more person-centred than its predecessor Reality Orientation, has also been shown to have benefit for people with dementia (Orrell *et al.* 2005). Sensory stimulation which includes engaging the senses through aromatherapy and/or massage (Ballard *et al.* 2002; Smallwood *et al.* 2001) or Snoozelen (e.g. Barker *et al.* 2003), is also popular. Other interventions include intergenerational programmes, which attempt to facilitate developmentally appropriate activities for people with dementia (Jarrott and Bruno 2003). Montessori-based methods, using materials to stimulate procedural memory or sensory stimulation, are tailored to individuals to help promote their well-being or functioning (Brenner and Brenner 2004; Camp and Skrajner 2004; Orsulic-Jeras, Judge and Camp 2000). The therapeutic use of dolls (Gibson 2005; James *et al.* 2005), the SPECAL approach (Garner 2004), horticultural therapy (Gigliotti, Jarrott and Yorgason 2004) and woodlands therapy (Pulsford, Rushforth and Connor 2000) are further examples. Developing a firm evidence base of what works for whom, when and in what setting is a difficult task. Given the heterogeneity of this population, the varied skill level of staff, the enormous variety of settings where activities take place alongside the problems of finding suitable outcome measures, it is not surprising that the research evidence for most of these activities appears weak (see reviews by Cohen-Mansfield 2005; Sherratt et al. 2004a; Thorgrimsen *et al.* 2004; Verkaik, Van Weert and Francke 2005). Nonetheless, from a practice perspective, seeing someone light up with delight when engaged in an activity that has meaning for them, is evidence enough that this is a worthwhile endeavour. It is applying occupation and activity as part of regular care practice that poses the real challenge.

Models of long-term care

Interventions are increasingly incorporating multiple components describing different aspects of care. Emotion-oriented care aims to help people cope with the emotional, cognitive and social consequences of living with dementia, and can encompass validation therapy (broadly validating subjective experience), reminiscence and sensory stimulation (Finnema *et al.* 2000). Integrated emotion-oriented care (which incorporates elements of emotion-oriented care into the 24-hour care of persons with dementia) was recently trialled in the Netherlands (Finnema *et al.* 2005).

Other examples of broadly person-centred approaches emphasise the importance of social support and networks for people with dementia such as the Best Friends approach (Bell and Troxell 1997), Alzheimer's cafes (Morrisey 2006) and

roups for people with dementia. The Enriched Oppor-
ogramme (Brooker and Woolley 2006) is an example
.. a multi-component initiative based on the principles of
person-centred care in nursing homes and extra-care housing,
and incorporating a specialist staff role – the 'Locksmith' whose
remit is to unlock the potential in all – an enriched activity
programme; individualised assessment; and staff training, development and management.

The person-centred care provider

Person-centred care is a term that has become common parlance
in dementia care. The ideas behind it no longer seem radical but
its practice is often ill-defined and difficult to evidence. The definition of person-centred care described within this book is a
four part composite. The basis for this is reviewed in Part 1. In
Part 2 I describe the VIPS Framework. The framework consists
of six key indicators for each of the VIPS elements. This can be
used for care providers to evidence their practice.

The VIPS framework is designed to help care providers
think through the issues in the provision of person-centred care
in a systematic way. Providing good quality person-centred care
is not an easy undertaking, particularly in a society that does not
value these services. It becomes more straightforward, however,
if we can articulate and clearly describe what it is we are doing as
dementia care providers to ensure that our services are person-
centred.

2

Valuing People

Element One of person-centred care is valuing people

Valuing people with dementia and those who care for them: promoting citizenship rights and entitlements regardless of age or cognitive impairment, and rooting out discriminatory practice.

Key indicators of valuing in care providers

- **VISION:** Is there a vision and mission statement about providing care that is person-centred?

- **HUMAN RESOURCE MANAGEMENT:** Are systems in place to ensure that staff feel valued by their employers?

- **MANAGEMENT ETHOS:** Are management practices empowering to staff delivering direct care?

- **TRAINING and STAFF DEVELOPMENT:** Are there systems in place to support development of a workforce skilled in person-centred care?

- **SERVICE ENVIRONMENTS:** Are there supportive and inclusive physical and social environments for people with cognitive disability?

- **QUALITY ASSURANCE:** Are Continuous Quality Improvement mechanisms in place that are driven by knowing and acting upon needs and concerns of service users?

People with dementia are part of every community in society. They are not confined to some distant place away from the rest of humanity. The stigma that surrounds dementia, however, means that the problems we all face about living with dementia, or caring for others with dementia, are often not talked about. People with dementia and those who care for them can become increasingly isolated, particularly as the disease progresses. We are, however, all citizens with all the rights that citizenship brings. We are also all human beings who depend on each other for love. People living with dementia are no less entitled to human rights or less in need of love.

Barriers to valuing

Most post-industrial societies are generally ageist. This means that people are discriminated against on the basis of age. Youth, and its stereotypes, are highly prized. By and large, older people are not valued unless they demonstrate that they are not stereotypically old. No one would say of an eight-year-old boy, 'Doesn't he look good for his age!', whereas this would be seen as a compliment for an 80-year-old. A cursory look at a nation's comedy TV programmes will give you a good gauge of the level of overt ageism in society. Certainly in the UK, older people are the target for jokes at their expense based on stereotypes that, if they were racial, would not be allowed to be broadcast.

In many post-industrial societies there are increasingly dispersed family networks and complicated family structures. Many countries are increasingly multi-cultural with many older people ageing in a second homeland. This means that caring directly for parents and grandparents is a real challenge. Providing good trans-cultural and multi-cultural care across generational boundaries is not easy either. The shifting age demographics mean that there are fewer young people in society and an increasing number living into very old age.

So, what we have is an increasing number of older people coupled with a decreasing resource to care properly. All prejudices increase when resources are scarce. As the balance between older people who need care increases and the numbers of younger people and resources available for care decreases, prejudice on the basis of age will increase.

Dementia is the most feared aspect of ageing. It is misunderstood by many, including many working in the caring professions. People with dementia suffer prejudice both because of their age and because of their intellectual decline. Stephen Post (Post 1995) described western society as hyper-cognitive. This is a special type of ageism, the victims of whom have cognitive impairment. There is also a prejudice about people with dementia because of the association with madness and psychiatric disorder that the label brings. The experience of many is that 'Dementia-ism' exists. It is related to other powerful prejudices such as sexism, racism and ageism but it also exists independently of all of these.

Services for people with dementia exist within society and those providing these services are subject to the same prejudice as the rest of society. Within care services for people who are elderly, or who have mental health problems, those who have dementia often appear to have to suffer even further prejudice. This discrimination is evident in service provision, resource allocation, research funding, media coverage, policy priorities, professional training and status, and the pay of care workers.

Within western philosophy, the question of what it is that defines a living creature as a 'person' has received considerable attention. Julian Hughes (2001) discusses various definitions of 'person'. Some philosophers see the definition of person as being dependent on consciousness of thought (being able to think about yourself thinking) and continuity of memory (being able to know your continuous life story). Using this definition would mean that an individual with dementia would not be seen as the same 'person' as their dementia progressed, because their continuous memory of themselves would change. At the most disabling stages of dementia, when consciousness of thinking is no longer evident, then 'the person' would cease to exist. Using this definition, as dementia destroys the brain, it also destroys the person. This fits well with the view of dementia propounded in the media as a living death that just leaves the body behind.

Hughes (2001) provides a philosophical argument for defining a person as a 'situated-embodied-agent' rather than relying on consciousness of thought for the definition. Defining the concept of person like this means that we should aspire to treat people with dementia at all stages of their disability in the way in which all people would wish to be treated. Similarly, Kitwood (1993a) described the person with dementia as:

> a person in the fullest sense: he or she is still an agent, one who can make things happen in the world, a sentient, relational and historical being (p.541).

Although these philosophical arguments may sometimes seem rather abstract to many people, the fact that these debates exist at all is an indicator of the lack of standing that people with dementia have. In 1986 in the UK, the King's Fund published *Living Well into Old Age*, which provided an explicit statement that people with dementia had the same rights and value as anyone else in society. The fact that an explicit statement had to be made at all is indicative that it was not a view universally held.

In Kitwood's writing, the ethical standing of people with dementia was discussed in terms of personhood: 'Personhood …carries essentially ethical connotations: to be a person is to have a certain status, to be worthy of respect' (Kitwood and Bredin 1992a, p.275). Likewise, John Bond (2001) describes personhood as 'all individuals are unique and have an absolute value…individuals do not function in isolation, they also have relationships with others; all human life is interconnected and interdependent' (p.47).

The lack of status and value that is attached to people with dementia also extends to those who want to look after their family members with dementia and those whose employment involves caring. Giving up paid employment to care for an elderly parent with dementia is not valued by society as much as staying at home to look after a terminally ill child. Likewise, the status afforded to a nurse working in a children's special care unit is much higher than the status of a nurse in an elderly care home.

Valuing the most vulnerable

On first contact, the moral and ethical basis for person-centred care is rather like 'mom and apple-pie'. In this day and age, how could anyone disagree that treating people struggling to live with dementia as whole human beings is the right and civilised way to respond? However, a cursory look around service provision, or a discussion with people with dementia and their families, suggests that people with dementia are not valued by society and the care they receive is not based on trust, respect and dignity.

In their recent report exploring the barriers to person-centred care for people living with dementia, Anthea Innes and colleagues (Innes, Macpherson and McCabe 2006) identified a lack of valuing by society of those employed to provide direct care, services being service-led rather than service user-led, and a workforce that felt undervalued, untrained and unsupported by their managers.

Standard One of the UK National Service Framework (NSF) (Department of Health 2001a) is about rooting out age discrimination. This is entirely laudable. However, it only addresses part of the prejudice for people with dementia. If their services are to be person-centred along with everybody else's, then dementia-ism needs to be rooted out with equal energy.

Person-centred care in the NSF is now established as central to policy on older people. There is a vested interest, however, from an economic point of view, in maintaining the position that people with dementia need very little in the way of skilled care interventions. In a political and economic context, where it appears that ever-increasing needs compete for a limited amount of resources, people with dementia are unlikely to ever be at the top of the list. The cause of promoting the rights of people with dementia does not make political sense.

Person-centred care is not generally the stuff of headline news. It will not attract votes. Occasionally, scandals hit the media but they usually focus on issues of physical abuse or malnourishment. These episodes are dreadful but not commonplace. Rather, most poor quality care and neglect that is experienced by people living with dementia is psychological rather than physical. Incomplete assessments, no one contacting you when they promised, feeling deceived, the withholding of information, the over-prescribing of drugs that you don't need and the under-prescribing of ones that you do. Lack of privacy, indignity, insensitivity, disrespect, stigmatisation, disempowerment and boredom are all very familiar features to service users and their families. The erosion of human and legal rights, and the overwhelming feeling that nothing personal is sacred, is still the day-to-day experience of people with dementia and their families. Government policy implementing a single assessment process will do little to change this. Although there are a greater number of older people in the electorate than ever before, those who are untouched personally by dementia are unlikely to put the needs of people with dementia at the top of their list for writing to their local MP. Generally, those who are fit and well find the spectre of dementia too distressing and would rather focus their energy elsewhere.

The personal is the political

Where does the will to provide person-centred care come from? Where do the champions and leaders of this cause come from? In the earlier section we saw that it is unlikely to be led at a government level. It is evident that things are changing, however. The rights of people with dementia are certainly more recognised than they were even five years ago.

In part, this is due to people with dementia speaking out for themselves. The practice of including people with dementia directly in the organisation of the Alzheimer's Society and Associations, and having people with dementia speak at national and international conferences, gives a very powerful message about the value of people with dementia in setting the agenda. However, those who are in long-term care are often too impaired and demoralised to be politically active. There are many excellent leaders in the dementia care field who have the experience of being a family carer. The strength of Alzheimer's societies and associations around the world bears witness to this. The rights of people with dementia to receive appropriate medication and care is clearly on the agenda, thanks in large part to the campaigning of the Alzheimer's Society in the UK and leaders from practice.

The question remains as to how can we change the face of long-term care for people with dementia to person-centred? Where is the leadership for this?

The answer, gentle reader, is that it comes from you.

In many respects, I am often surprised that many services for people with dementia manage to operate in a way that is valuing of people with dementia. Fortunately, there have always been a good number of people who have operated with compassion and basic common-sense in their human relationships, even before we had any literature on person-centred care. There is a strong desire on an individual level from many people to provide health and social care that enables people to live their lives to the full. Sometimes this desire comes from family experience. Often it comes from a powerful drive for social justice and inclusion. There is also an increasing recognition that working with people with dementia is a skilled undertaking and that it can be a very rewarding area of work.

In recognition of the fact that it is unlikely that there will be a political sea change in supporting the rights of people with dementia, being proactive in promoting the rights of this group has to be part of the definition of person-centred care. Unless we, as care providers, practitioners, researchers and family members, promote the value of the people we care for and their rights to be treated as equal citizens, then we collude with the political expedient that these people do not really matter. Unless we let those in power know that this is a skilled area of work that cannot be done successfully on the cheap by staff with no training, then we are devaluing the lives of those we care for. If we devalue a person, then this is not person-centred care.

Organisations that value people

If we encourage dementia care practitioners to adopt a person-centred approach without addressing the larger organisational context, we are setting them up to fail. The practice of caring for very vulnerable people with dementia in large groups with low staffing levels can place care workers in an intolerable bind when trying to provide person-centred care. How to balance the needs of one individual who requires lots of attention against the needs of the wider group, who may be equally needy but make less show of it, is one that faces dementia care practitioners, day in day out.

If a care organisation is to deliver person-centred care in anything but a non-trivial manner, the rights of all people regardless of age and cognitive ability has to be driven from the top down. It is the top-level leadership within a care organisation that determines this. The person-centred approach is an ethical code that encompasses all relationships. This includes not just people with dementia but those of us who work in this area and those who are family carers. It is a code that values all people as unique individuals, tries to see things from the viewpoint of the other and recognises the interdependence of us all.

The person-centred approach is about the building of authentic relationships. Organisations that adopt a person-centred approach to care also recognise the need to work by the same set of principles with their staff. If the personhood of an individual member of staff is not respected, then she or he in turn will find it difficult to maintain respect for those she or he cares for over a sustained period of time.

Direct care workers for older people are one of the lowest paid groups in health and social care, often working in poor conditions with high risk of injury (Noelker and Ejaz 2005). Staff turnover is high, and the quality of training and supervision is generally poor. The way in which direct care workers are treated has a direct impact on the care they provide. Empowering direct care staff through adequate induction and training is a crucial first step towards improving the lived experience of care for people with dementia.

Rather than seeing people with dementia as the ones having problems and those who are caring having none, Kitwood suggested that many of the problems experienced in dementia care are interpersonal. They occur in the communication. He suggests we need to view the relationships between 'carers' and 'cared for' as psychotherapeutic relationships and, in this respect just as in psychotherapeutic work, the helpers need to be aware of their own issues around caring for others.

In person-centred care, the relationships between all people in the care environment should be nurtured.

> I believe that people with dementia are making an important journey from cognition, through emotion, into spirit. I've begun to realise what really remains throughout this journey is what is really important, and what disappears is what is not important. I think that if society could appreciate this, then people with dementia would be respected and treasured. (Bryden 2005, p.159)

Valuing people is at the heart of person-centred care. If this element of the definition is not made explicit in value statements, training, staff selection, standards, policies and procedures, then services will not maintain a person-centred approach for long.

Putting valuing into practice

The indicators in the Valuing People element of VIPS primarily need to be led by those managing the care organisation. These indicators are about the organisational vision and culture and how these are then set out in various organisational operating procedures.

As managers and leaders within social care, it sometimes feels that all we can do is to struggle to find the resources to meet minimum standards of basic physical care. Working within cash constraints, dealing with staff shortages, and being the repository for everyone's complaints and guilt grinds leaders down over time. It diminishes the personhood of those in leadership positions. It means that those of us who are responsible for setting the value base for an organisation often feel devalued ourselves. If you are in a senior position in a care organisation, you will recognise this only too well.

Providing person-centred care that values all people is in itself a journey. The fact that you are reading this book means that you have already begun this journey. What follows are a series of questions to help your organisation reflect on where you are in terms of the Valuing People element of person-centred care.

The questions that follow all relate to valuing. I outline why each question is important in providing person-centred care and how care providers might collect evidence to know how to answer the questions posed.

---

1. Vision

Is there a vision and mission statement about providing care that is person-centred?

An organisation's mission statement spells out its reason for being and its purpose. Valuing people has to begin at the top. Valuing the equality of all regardless of age and cognitive disability is a challenge that is difficult to achieve. It is impossible to achieve fully unless those at board or trustee level take it as underpinning all their decisions. Agreeing this in its vision or mission statement means that the organisation is making public its policy of promoting the rights of people with dementia.

Developing a mission statement is an exercise in setting the value base of an organisation. It has to involve all the key stakeholders if it is to be owned and abided by. Management textbooks devote significant space to advice on developing mission statements.

Written material about the service should be provided in a way that is accessible to all service users. This includes a vision statement about people being supported by the service regardless of their age or level of cognitive ability, and how this is achieved. This information should also be available in spoken and other formats where appropriate. This purpose should be clear to all members of staff at all levels from direct care to board level. It should be clear to service users, their families and all who come into contact with the service.

This is a fairly straightforward indicator to provide evidence for. Mission statements are fairly prominent on the publicity material of most organisations. This can be evidenced by an audit of materials available to service users about the service.

Whether the principles enshrined in mission statements actually guide the priorities within decision making is another matter. Interviewing key managers or questions relating to the guiding principles in decision making may help to provide this.

---

2. Human resource management

Are systems in place to ensure that staff feel valued by their employers?

If an organisation values people for their inherent worth as human beings, then it will seek to fight discrimination of all sorts. Are people from all walks of life welcome? This is part of person-centred care for staff. If the staff group feel valued, then they in turn are likely to value those they care for. This should be reflected in practices that affect recruitment, promotion, pay and conditions, and that reward skills and expertise in person-centred care. How are complaints managed? This will be evidenced from personnel practice, from an analysis of the workforce profile and also from staff surveys and interviews.

If staff are to see communication, integrity and nurturing as important in their work with people with dementia, then this should be their experience of how the organisation relates to them as workers. Is there a recognition of the importance of building teams that work well together and who are united in their purpose? Teams that see value in working together are more likely to promote a sense of shared community with all the service users in their facility, with less risk of scapegoating those people who do not fit in easily. Is there a whistle-blowing policy? How is sickness managed? What sort of induction, appraisal and reward systems exist? What are the terms and conditions of employment?

How is workplace stress managed? Providing person-centred dementia care is emotionally labour intensive. How is it identified when a team is in need of extra support? What form does extra support take? How is it accessed? How is it reviewed? Is there a system of debriefing and reflection following particularly stressful events?

This can be evidenced by staff surveys, focus groups and interviews, policy and procedures audit, and external accreditation such as Investors in People.

---

3. Management ethos

Are management practices empowering to staff delivering direct care?

Providing person-centred care for people with dementia often relies on taking advantage of opportunities as they occur. Staff who feel their ideas for good practice are met with enthusiasm are more likely to react positively to ideas and challenges from service users. If a 'can do' culture exists for staff, they are more likely to promote this with service users and families.

Markers of this might include clear avenues for communication that are used frequently between different levels of the organisation. How are decisions made and disseminated throughout the organisation? Staff who feel that they understand why decisions have been taken, and are knowledgeable about the process, are surely more likely to keep families and service users better informed in a way that deals with issues rather than apportions blame for bad decisions to the powers that be.

Is there a consultation process that is trusted throughout the organisation? Staff who feel that they have been consulted over practice are more likely to institute consultation practices with families and service users. Is there an 'open door' management practice? Staff who feel that they can approach their managers if they have a problem that they cannot resolve, or an idea that will improve practice, are more likely to encourage and listen to ideas from families and service users. Is there delegation of resource management to the optimum level to provide person-centred care?

Without the ability to communicate effectively with each other, the basis for providing an adequate social environment is flawed. In the absence of good communication, paranoia, confusion and anxiety flourish. This is true both for staff teams and for people in care.

How are matters communicated between members of staff? Is adequate time provided for handovers and communal problem-solving? Who talks to whom? What is the communication like within a shift? What is the communication like between front-line and senior staff? What is communication like between shifts, between night and day staff, between staff working in different sections of the same building? Is the communication two-way? Do people feel listened to and have the chance to have their say?

This can be evidenced through staff surveys, focus groups and interviews, and audits of staff meetings. High levels of complaints from families can be an indicator that communication has broken down at a fundamental level.

---

4. Training and staff development

Are there systems in place to support development of a workforce skilled in person-centred care?

Maintaining person-centred care over time for people with dementia is not an easy or trivial process. Dementia services do not have a tradition of skilled care and the practices that are required to maintain it. There should be a recognition in your organisation that caring for people with dementia is skilled work that is emotionally and physically labour intensive. What is the training and education strategy? What is available at induction regarding working with people with dementia? How are training needs identified? What specialist courses are available? How is learning supported in the workplace? What is the level of expertise of more senior people? Have they got accredited qualifications in gerontology or dementia studies?

Are there opportunities for reflective practice, supervision and mentoring? When individual practitioners or staff teams are feeling out of their depth working with a particular service user or family, how is more expert help accessed?

This can be evidenced by staff surveys and interviews, training records, evaluation of training and skills analysis. It can also be tracked in critical incident analysis to see whether training is identified as a significant factor.

---

5. Service environments

Are there supportive and inclusive physical and social environments for people with cognitive disability?

Once an organisation has taken on board the need to eradicate anti-discriminatory practice against people with dementia, the next stage is to look at the active steps it takes to support people with dementia. If an organisation is able to provide examples of providing individualised care, taking seriously the viewpoint of people with dementia and providing a supportive social psychology, as outlined in other chapters in this book, then it is likely they are serious about their commitment to anti-discriminatory practice.

Anti-discriminatory practice means that people with dementia have the same rights as everyone else. It does not mean that people with dementia do not need extra help in everyday life. For example, we would expect that those in wheelchairs have a right to enter buildings, and we would provide elevators or ramps to help them achieve this. Likewise, we would expect that a person with dementia has the right to find their way around the building with clear signage and way-finding markers.

At a corporate level, that means that there should be evidence that this is taken into consideration in design briefs for buildings, and fixtures and fittings. In the general physical design, are features such as clear colours, way-finding memory markers, unambiguous surfaces to walk on, easy access to a safe outdoor environment, natural light, low numbers of blind corners, no obvious locked doors and unobtrusive use of technology maximised to provide a non-confusing and low anxiety-provoking physical environment?

At a corporate level, there should also be recognition that all staff coming into contact with service users with dementia should understand some of the special needs around communication. Is it policy that all staff having direct service-user contact are aware of how to help someone with dementia feel at ease? Is this evidenced in staff induction and training?

This can be evidenced by service users' interviews and surveys; family and supporters' interviews and surveys; physical environment audits; training records; skills analysis and observation of practice.

---

6. Quality assurance

Are Continuous Quality Improvement mechanisms in place that are driven by knowing and acting upon needs and concerns of service users?

Knowing how service users feel about the service th
on an ongoing basis is central to person-centred care. 1
your organisation know and act upon the views of servi
Does it undertake regular satisfaction surveys, interview, ⌐cus
groups, reference groups or observation of practice such as Dementia Care Mapping (DCM)? Are the views of all service users
regardless of level of cognitive impairment taken into account in
this process, or just the most vocal?

Involving service users and knowing their views is central to
person-centred care – or any customer care activity. In the
dementia care field, this can take place through residents'
groups, carers' groups, user forums and other ad hoc reference
groups. How are these organised? How often do they occur?
Whose responsibility are they? What happens to the views or
decisions made at these meetings? Are they seen as central to the
decision-making process, or are they just an add-on?

This can be evidenced by service users' and carers' interviews and surveys; audits of quality procedures and meetings;
results of quality surveys and reviews; external quality assurance
accreditation; training records; skills analysis and observation of
practice.

Summary
Element One of person-centred care is about valuing people
throughout the care organisation. If staff do not feel valued by
the organisation they work for, then it is unlikely they will be
able to sustain valuing and caring relationships with people with
dementia over a sustained period. Valuing people can be seen in
many organisational processes around communication, anti-
discriminatory practice, human resources management, training,
operational management, consultation and quality management.

3

Individualised Care

> ### Element Two of person-centred care is treating people as individuals
>
> Treating people as individuals: appreciating that all people have a unique history and personality, physical and mental health, and social and economic resources, and that these will affect their response to dementia.

Key indicators of individualised care in care providers

- **CARE PLANNING:** Do you identify strengths and vulnerabilities across a wide range of needs, and have individualised care plans that reflect a wide range of strengths and needs?

- **REGULAR REVIEWS:** Are individual care plans reviewed on a regular basis?

- **PERSONAL POSSESSIONS:** Do service users have their own personal clothing and possessions for everyday use?

- **INDIVIDUAL PREFERENCES:** Are individual likes and dislikes, preferences and daily routines known about by direct care staff and acted upon?

- **LIFE HISTORY:** Are care staff aware of individual life histories and key stories of proud times, and are these used regularly?

- **ACTIVITY AND OCCUPATION:** Are there a variety of activities available to meet the needs and abilities of all service users?

The most concrete implication of person-centred care, which sometimes becomes its whole definition, is about taking an individualised approach to assessing and meeting the needs of people with dementia. This element of the definition encompasses all those ways of working that consider men and women with all their individual strengths and vulnerabilities, and sees their dementia as part of that picture rather than defining their identity. This approach again has resonance with the work of Carl Rogers for whom each client was a unique and whole person.

Linda Clare and colleagues also see focusing on the richness and uniqueness of each individual as important: 'Dementia is more than simply a matter of brain decay. People contribute a unique personality and a set of life experiences, coping resources and social networks' (Clare *et al.* 2003, p.251).

Likewise, Graham Stokes (Stokes 2000) takes the uniqueness of individuals as a major part of his definition of person-centred care. He expands this model in a very practical way to work with people with dementia, who are in distress, by understanding the uniqueness of each person. Mary Marshall takes a slightly different emphasis: '[Person-centred care] means, in brief, that care is tailored to meet the needs of the individual rather than the group or the needs of the staff' (Marshall 2001, p.175).

Inherent in this view is that the person with dementia is the focus, and not the group into which professionals and staff might place them.

Is individualised care planning person-centred care?

The UK National Service Framework (NSF) chose to focus on the Individualised Care element of person-centred care. The aim within this standard in the NSF is about treating people as individuals and providing them with packages of care that meet their individual needs. In the more detailed Department of Health Guidance, *Everybody's Business: Integrated Mental Health Services for Older Adults*, again the emphasis is on person-centred care planning: '[care planning] supports the person to be as independent as possible in aspects of daily living but is also sensitive to meeting the needs of their disability by providing personal support when required' (DH 2005, p.31).

It then becomes similar to the term 'patient-centred care' or 'resident-focused care', which is also sometimes used interchangeably with person-centred care. If the intention is solely to look at a person's needs in the context of their being a patient or a resident, then it is probably clearer to use the term 'individualised patient care' or 'individualised resident care'. In Germany, the term 'patientenzentriert' – 'patient centred' has existed for many years and is used with respect to care in hospitals. Likewise the term 'patient-centred' is used frequently in the UK, the USA and Australia.

Although this is clearly linked to the Individualised Care element of person-centred care it provides a narrower focus than person-centred care, in that the person can only express those individual needs that are covered by being a patient. Those working in the care professions can become so conditioned by defining people they work with by their diagnostic group, problem type or service need, that they are at risk of overlooking the person behind the label. For example a patient might be able to have an individualised plan of continence care but not be able to help make a cup of tea, because the risk is too great for the hospital's insurers. The person in this context is defined by their status as a patient having continence needs, rather than an appreciation of their need to maintain a lifelong activity such as tea making.

There is a danger that, by just focusing on individualised care, the person with dementia stays firmly hidden behind their disease label and person-centred care still does not occur. Although it is not possible to do person-centred care without taking an individualised approach, it is possible to do individualised care that is not person-centred. Inserting a problem focus into individualised care can make it difficult to continue to see the person as an individual in the round.

Person-centred individualised care

Kitwood (1990a, 1990b) characterised dementia as a dialectical interplay between neurological impairment, the psychological make-up of the individual with dementia and the social context (social psychology) in which they find themselves. This later became the Enriched Model of dementia, incorporating the biological, the psychological and the social aspects of a care environment which is summarised in Table 3.1.

The equation in Table 3.1 aids understanding of the unique position of each person with dementia. Every such person will have a different pattern of neurological impairment, a different health profile, a unique history and personality, and a unique interplay of all these in the social aspects of their current situation. It is a person-centred model rather than a biological model and has many uses in assessment and care practice. Hazel May and Paul Edwards (May and Edwards, in press) have used this equation as a framework for care planning.

Table 3.1: The Enriched Model of dementia

Dementia = NI + H + B + P + SP	
NI =	Neurological impairment
H =	Health and physical fitness
B =	Biography – life history
P =	Personality
SP =	Social psychology

Neurological impairment (NI)

The neurological impairment associated with dementia affects memory function, the ability to use and understand spoken and written language, the ability to carry out practical everyday tasks, the ability to perceive the world as others do, and the ability to plan a course of action and to see things from other people's viewpoints. These impairments are quite subtle and easy to misunderstand at first, but become more obvious as the dementia progresses over time. Being aware of the manifestation of these impairments is a key element of good dementia care in enabling care workers to respond appropriately. The aim is to find a response that supports the person with dementia while not undermining their remaining abilities.

Common cognitive impairments in dementia, such as poor learning of new information, dysphasias, dyspraxias and visuo-perceptual deficits, mean that people with dementia will interpret their social and physical environments in a unique way. If these interpretations of the environment are not understood and compensated for, then the person with dementia will experience excess disability. All too often, however, this is attributed to neurological impairment rather than as a function of an unsupportive care environment (Stokes 2000).

Health and physical fitness (H)

When someone is elderly, and particularly if they have the label of dementia, there is a tendency for family carers, care staff and professionals to attribute any increase in confused behaviour to the dementia. However, people with dementia are also much more susceptible to acute confusional states and delirium arising from physical health problems such as urinary or chest infections, constipation, hormonal imbalances, dehydration, malnutrition, over-medication and sedation. This is compounded further by the fact that some people with dementia will not be able to give an accurate account of their symptoms because of their memory problems. For example, if a person with dementia is unable to remember that they have been experiencing chest pains, they are unlikely to seek help for their symptoms. It then becomes incumbent on those delivering care to be extra vigilant regarding changes in physical health status.

Biography or life history (B)

People make sense of what is happening to them in the here and now by reference to experiences they have had in the past. Because of the type of brain damage they have, the more recent past for people with dementia has often not been laid down reliably within memory stores. People with dementia who are in a nursing home, for example, may have very little understanding of where they are. First, they may not remember anything about the admission process because of memory loss and, second, nursing homes do not relate to any past experiences they have.

Nonetheless, people with dementia will try to make sense of where they are. For some, the nursing home may look rather like their former workplace in particular elements. Knowledge of someone's work history may help staff to understand so-called confused behaviour. For example, people who have held managerial positions during their working life may find it very confusing to be told what to do by a care worker who, in their eyes, is a junior employee, particularly if what they are being told to do relates to personal care activities. Likewise, if a person with dementia thinks she is a care worker's mother and the care worker is attempting to help take her to the toilet, she is likely to get irritated and confused. A man who all his life has had to milk cows at 4am may become very distressed at being told that he cannot.

Past experiences of institutional care are particularly important to know about. For example:

A person who is the ex-matron of a nursing home is likely to want to sit in the office and check through the medical notes or duty roster and will not take kindly to being told that she may not do so by someone she considers her junior staff.

A person who has spent time in an orphanage or a prison at an earlier time of their life may interpret particular staff actions in ways that were not intended by those staff members.

Personality (P)

This refers to the totality of the strengths and vulnerabilities that we all carry with us as human beings, and that will have a direct effect on how an individual copes with the effects of their dementia. If a person has always placed great value on being in control of their lives and what happens around them, they are likely to struggle more with the consequences of dementia than someone who has always been happy to leave decisions to someone else. An extrovert may cope better with communal living than an introvert. Personality does not usually change as a result of having dementia. The ways in which people respond to stress and challenge are well-learnt behaviours. Talking to family members and friends about how people have coped with stress and adversity, and what has helped them through it, can offer clues to how they can best be assisted to cope with the challenges that living with dementia brings.

Social psychology (SP)

This is the social and psychological environment in which people with dementia find themselves. Primarily it is about the relationships between people. Kitwood's view of person-centred care for people with dementia was that it took place in the context of relationships. He wrote a great deal about this and the way in which social psychology could be supportive or damaging to people with dementia. As verbal abilities are lost, the importance of warm, accepting human contact through non-verbal channels becomes even more important than before.

With the onset of dementia, individuals are very vulnerable to their psychological defences being radically attacked and broken down. As the sense of self breaks down, it becomes increasingly important that it is held within the relationships that the person with dementia experiences. These relationships cannot be developed through the traditional therapy hour as in person-centred psychotherapy. Rather, the development of relationships occurs through the day-to-day interactions.

The individual experience of dementia will be determined in part by the social environment. Much can be done to ensure that the social environment is generally supportive of the needs of people with dementia. I return to this in greater depth in Chapter 5. When trying to determine an individualised plan of care, however, the way in which people respond to their surroundings and what triggers positive or negative reactions is important to assess.

Putting individualised care into practice

What follows is a series of questions to help your organisation reflect on where you are in terms of the Individualised Care element of person-centred care.

The indicators in the Individualised Care element of VIPS primarily need to be led by those setting the clinical or care standards within the care organisation. These indicators are about the processes that operate to ensure that care is delivered to a high standard.

As leaders for care standards within health and social care, sometimes it feels that all we can do is to keep the standards safe and prevent adverse events. Ensuring that health and safety and statutory legislation is met, keeping up with the latest developments, reporting on every activity imaginable means that clinical leaders often feel overwhelmed by the level of demands upon them. If you are in a senior position in a care organisation, you will recognise this only to well.

Providing person-centred care that really takes individualised care seriously is a tough challenge. It is easy to skim the surface when it comes to the lives of people with dementia. The fact that you are reading this chapter means that you take this endeavour seriously and have a desire not to just skim the surface.

The questions that follow relate to these key areas. I outline why they are of importance to person-centred care and how you might collect evidence to know how to answer the questions posed.

---

1. Care planning

Do you identify strengths and vulnerabilities across a wide range of needs, and have individualised care plans that reflect a wide range of strengths and needs?

Individualised assessment and analysis sets a basis from which interventions can be designed for both enhancing well-being by appropriately matching activity and occupation to persons with dementia, or reducing disturbed mood or behaviour. Many other interacting factors are likely to require taking into consideration, such as level of dependency and a range of socio-economic, gender, ethnic or cultural differences.

Using Kitwood's Enriched Model of dementia, discussed earlier, is a good place to start in ensuring that you are covering a wide range of needs. The person-centred care planning templates (May and Edwards, in press) provide an excellent basis for this. They identify Biography, Personality, Lifestyle, Life at the moment, Health and Cognitive support needs, and Capacity for Doing as key domains.

In the Enriched Opportunities Programme (Brooker, Woolley and Lee, in press), four different domains were addressed for each individual to help identify ways of optimising the well-being of individuals living in long-term care.

The first domain was cognitive ability and engagement capacity: How does this person think? How do they communicate? How do they relate to the world? How do they relate to objects? This helps in planning the level that a person can engage with activities and what type of support they will need.

The second domain was life history: What are experiences from the person's past that could hold clues to improving and maintaining well-being now? This provides information as to what activities will be familiar and enjoyed. It also identifies objects that could trigger positive memories and actions. This involved the completion of life story books and life boxes, either completed with the person themselves or sometimes with the help of family members.

The third domain was personality: What is this person like? What motivates them? What influences their mood? This provides clues as to what the person enjoys and doesn't enjoy. This was completed through observations and by discussion with the key worker and family.

The final area was an assessment of current interests: What happens in the home that brings this person to life? What delights them? This provides the establishment of everyday opportunities that can bring real joy. This was completed through observations and by discussion with the key worker and family.

Evidencing whether individualised assessments take place, and whether these are used in care planning, can usually be seen from a case note audit. Ensuring that what has been learnt from the assessment is known about and is used in practice, will often only be accessible through interviewing staff or from observation of practice. Tracking an individual service user through their initial assessment and care planning can be particularly illuminating.

---

2. Regular reviews

Are individual care plans reviewed on a regular basis?

The needs of people with dementia change over time. This is true for all of us, but particularly when working with progressive conditions we can be sure that change will occur. The pace of change will vary on an individual basis. For some the pace will be slow and insidious, so much so that it is easy to overlook subtle problems that may be causing a sense of failure in the person with dementia. For this reason, it is important that there is a fail-safe procedure so that everyone's care plan gets looked at, at least every six months to ensure that it is still meeting needs. On the other hand, there will be people whose needs change very quickly either because of the nature of their dementia or because of some other unstable physical health condition. Structures should be in place so that care plans can be reviewed quickly when necessary.

Building good relationships with local mental health teams or specialist services can help ensure that health and well-being is maintained at the optimal level. They can be useful where there are issues of significant deterioration, worsening confusion or depression.

Evidence of the effectiveness of the review process can be gained through a care plan audit and a review of procedures surrounding the updating and review of care plans. Ensuring that what is in the care plan is actually used in practice will often only be accessible through interviewing staff, from observation of practice or through case tracking.

---

3. Personal possessions

Do service users have their own personal clothing and possessions for everyday use?

As dementia progresses, people will obtain much greater comfort from wearing clothes that look familiar and using objects that are well known, rather than getting to grips with new possessions. The reasons for this are two-fold. First, familiar items are a touchstone in a world that feels increasingly alien to people living with dementia. They link the present with the past, the unfamiliar with the known. Second, as dementia progresses, people often lose the ability to learn how to use new objects quickly, whereas with old objects the patterns are well learnt. Most of us have the experience of turning on a lamp with which we are familiar without even consciously thinking about where the switch is. With a new lamp we have to stop and think. It is the latter action that becomes difficult to manage in dementia. Surround the person with things that are familiar and they will be more at ease. When new things need to be purchased, try to buy the same make or model, or buy clothes in the same material as ones that were cherished.

If the care organisation provides residential care, the procedures surrounding the bringing in of personal possessions and
furniture can provide evidence of how seriously this is taken.
Involving families and friends in buying new clothes can help
ensure continuity if the person is not able to actively participate.

This can be evidenced by service users' and carers' interviews and surveys; observation of practice; assessment and care
plan audit; Individual Care Pathways and case tracking.

---

4. Individual preferences

Are individual likes and dislikes, preferences and daily
routines, known about by direct care staff and acted
upon?

If familiar objects are important in dementia care, then familiar
foods, drinks, music and routines are even more so. Familiarity
with day-to-day experiences help to establish security, trust and
comfort. As anxiety decreases, so will the likelihood that a person will try to 'go home' in an attempt to find the familiar.

Helping staff to recognise the importance of this is central to
raising their empathy with their clients. In a staff training
session,[1] it can be useful to get staff to describe their morning
routine to each other – what time do they rise? Are they the first
up? Do they get dressed before breakfast? What jobs do they do
first thing? What do they eat and drink? Do they sit with others?
Cook for others? Do they wash? Shower? Read the paper?
Listen to the radio? Watch TV? People are always amazed at the
variety even in a group who all work in a similar sort of job. I
then ask them to imagine that, instead of their own routine, they

---

1   Special thanks to my colleague Dee Westwood for first describing
      this training exercise to me, which I have used many times since.

had to follow someone else's in the room. They have no choice as to whom and they have to follow it. I explain that this might be a parallel with being admitted to a nursing home. How does this make them feel? What would they miss the most?

There is an increasing recognition that trying to ensure there is familiarity in long-held routines and preferences is an important way of helping people feel at ease. Sometimes people will be able to tell us about these routines and preferences for themselves. Other times, they will not, which is when getting this information from family and friends can be useful. Again, ensuring that direct care staff know about these routines and preferences and use them every day can be difficult. I have lost count of the number of 'student projects' I have known about where students of one profession or another have collated this sort of information only for it to be filed away in a filing cabinet and never to make an impact on people's lives.

However, keeping to routines and well-known preferences does not necessarily mean that things have to be the same every day. People will be willing to try something new as they always were – and perhaps more so in some cases. It is important for staff to observe body language and reactions to new situations; to know what it is that works in the here and now.

People with dementia are very vulnerable to feeling culturally isolated. If any of us are feeling vulnerable, then familiar touchstones of our cultural identity, our spirituality or religion, and food and drinks and music with which we are familiar are likely to have a calming effect. Vulnerability, anxiety and alienation are more likely to increase if those elements are missing. Because the person with dementia lacks the internal resources and reasoning to protect themselves against alienation, this can be much more damaging to their sense of self than it would be if they had intact cognitive abilities.

This can be evidenced by service users' and carers' interviews and surveys; observation of practice; assessment and care plan audit; Individual Care Pathways and case tracking.

> ## 5. Life history
>
> Are care staff aware of individual life histories and key stories of proud times, and are these used regularly?

As dementia progresses, it becomes more difficult to hold on to the stories of one's life and to be able to tell others of the defining moments that shaped our identity. One of the jobs of caring for someone with dementia is to learn these key stories and hold this narrative for them. This can be used to improve self-esteem and to maintain an identity in the face of increasing confusion. As the capacity for engagement becomes more difficult, objects that trigger good feelings become increasingly important. In the Enriched Opportunities Programme we used 'life boxes' that contained cherished objects. This was more meaningful to many than life-story books or even photo albums:

> The life boxes help don't they because they've all got something in their life box. So we've learned new stuff where they've got… And that's good if you're on a different House Group and residents you're not familiar with or…they are quite helpful. (Residential care worker)

Past experiences of vulnerability and trauma, particularly those that happened in childhood or teenage years can often be relived during a dementia illness which may have emotional resonance with these past experiences. If someone has a history of being sexually abused, they may find help with personal care activities particularly traumatic.

Understanding a person's past history is crucial to providing person-centred care for people with dementia. This can be evidenced around looking at procedures for how key stories are known about and how these are communicated. Some of this can be seen by assessment and care plan audit. Knowing whether they are used by staff in everyday situations requires observation of practice.

---

6. Activity and occupation

Are there a variety of activities available to meet the needs and abilities of all service users?

Boredom and lack of meaningful activity is rife in institutional care for older people generally, but particularly those with dementia who often find it difficult to initiate or sustain activities. Finding things that interest and sustain people can be a challenge. As well as knowing what is meaningful to each individual, understanding the capabilities of individuals with regard to their level or severity of dementia is likely to be important for providing suitable activities. In the early stages, cognitive therapies or goal-directed activities such as competitive games or crafts might be most productive. Behavioural interventions or creative therapies might be most therapeutic in the middle stages of dementia while sensory stimulation might be most appropriate for people with the highest levels of cognitive and functional impairment (Cheston 1998; Perrin and May 1999).

How this can be achieved in long-term care settings or by people living with dementia at home requires careful consideration. Who has responsibility for ensuring that service users have access to fun and meaningful activity on a day-to-day basis? How is this provided? How is it monitored to ensure it meets the needs of individuals?

Activity organisers or co-ordinators are employed by some residential care providers to try to meet these needs for occupation. In the USA, Canada and Australia, the role of 'Recreational Therapist' has been developed. In the Enriched Opportunities Programme the specialist role of 'Locksmith' was developed in order to meet this need in nursing homes and extra care housing. In any institutional service setting, there has to be an appreciation that all staff from direct care workers through to management share in the responsibility for the provision of fun and occupation that gives meaning and structure to life and staves off boredom.

In the Enriched Opportunities Programme, one of the keys was to find individualised simple and fun activities that could occur every day. Although the locksmith assessed what worked with whom and communicated it to all the team, it was the regular care staff who carried it out on a one-to-one basis or in small groups. The shift manager had to give priority to this in workload planning and scheduling. The key was usually finding something simple and straightforward that could be incorporated into everyday care as the following quotes from locksmiths and residential care workers illustrate:

> Warm water, warm soapy water – dip their hands in there, they were just…they don't go for longer than about ten minutes. That is very soothing, it calms them down… concentrating on that, at the end of it.

> We have one woman that spends a lot of time in the rooms, and we know from her family that she used to listen to classical music. Now because we're playing that a lot, this lady, we're getting so much more response. She's smiling, she's happy, she's laughing. And we haven't had that for a long time – and it's lovely. It's really lovely.

> We've actually got a bottle of Tia Maria in there for her as well, and sherry, so she's having a tipple with her meals, and it's lovely – she enjoys it. And her chocolate. So even though we're not doing a LOT with her down here in the main lounge, she is getting more one-to-one attention. She's getting something she likes listening to, she likes a drink, and a lot of touchy-feely.

> With Elsie who's so difficult to engage… With the balloons, she loves knocking balloons around. I mean she's just like plus 5, plus 5, plus 5 (exceptional well-being). And once you stop knocking it around she'll kind of hold on to a balloon and use it in a sensory way, so it's brilliant.

> It is the simple things, it is like last week they had a snowball and put it in front of Bill (resident) and he picked it up and was passing it round, that is an activity. It is sensory, it's…whereas if somebody comes in and says you bake a cake what reaction are you going to get?

Involving outside therapists, entertainers and volunteers is a further way in which the environment can be enriched. In the Enriched Opportunities Programme, this was led by the locksmith but it was also recognised that the staff team and the management had their part to play here too. Some of the observations the residential care workers picked up are as follows:

> I think the pat dog works well with those that like dogs. They get a lot out of that. And that's quite a nice one as well isn't it, you know, if somebody's coming in to do it.

> I know there are a couple on three that like their own space and what have you and I have noticed that they…they don't need any cajoling or anything to come up now.

> They will say 'oooh what's it…?'

> Because one of them says now…'oh the lady is here'. And they come straight up and like they are all together rather than sitting.

> And like aromatherapy. They enjoy it.

> On St Patrick's Day we had two Irish Dance girls in and the reaction from some of the residents was lovely. And we did a proper Irish meal and oh it was really nice. The relatives came in and they enjoyed it – the residents enjoyed it.

> They love live action stuff – close stuff.

This can be evidenced by service users' and carers' interviews and surveys; observation of practice; assessment and care plan audit; Individual Care Pathways and case tracking. Interviews with staff and families and with service users will reveal how people feel about the level and types of day-to-day activity a service can provide. It will also be evident in observation of practice. In residential care, a Dementia Care Mapping (DCM) evaluation can demonstrate whether a good provision of activity and occupation is present that is appropriate for the service users. This would be evidenced by a diverse range of Behavioural Category Codes and in relatively high levels of mood and engagement resulting in a positive Well-being score across the day.

Summary

Element Two of person-centred care is about providing care on an individualised basis where people are known about and accepted in their entirety – not just because of their diagnostic label. The degree to which organisations treat people as individuals can be seen in many organisational processes around assessment and care planning. It is also evident in how people lead their day-to-day lives, and whether this is based around their lifestyles, preferences and needs for activity and occupation.

4

Personal Perspectives

Element Three of person-centred care is looking at the world from the perspective of the person with dementia

Looking at the world from the perspective of the person with dementia: recognising that each person's experience has its own psychological validity, that people with dementia act from this perspective, and that empathy with this perspective has its own therapeutic potential.

Key indicators for care providers of taking the perspective of the person with dementia

- **COMMUNICATION WITH SERVICE USERS:** On a day-to-day basis, are service users asked for their preferences, consent and opinions?

- **EMPATHY AND ACCEPTABLE RISK:** Do staff show the ability to put themselves in the position of the person they are caring for and to think about decisions from their point of view?

- **PHYSICAL ENVIRONMENT:** Is the physical environment – e.g. noise, temperature – managed on a day-to-day basis to help people with dementia feel at ease?

- **PHYSICAL HEALTH:** Are the physical health needs of people with dementia, including pain assessment, sight and hearing problems, given due attention?

- **CHALLENGING BEHAVIOUR AS COMMUNICATION:** Is 'challenging behaviour' analysed to discover the underlying reasons for it?

- **ADVOCACY:** In situations where the actions of an individual with dementia are at odds with the safety and well-being of others, how are the rights of the individual protected?

Person-centred care is part of the phenomenological school of psychology. In this, the subjective experience of the individual is seen as reality. The starting point for helping someone is trying to understand the world as they see it. Rogerian person-centred therapeutic approaches would see entering the frame of reference of the individual and understanding the world from their point of view as key to working therapeutically. Part of taking the perspective of the person with dementia as a starting point for care is the ability to relate to them directly, seeing them as a fellow human being.

Naomi Feil's validation therapy takes entering the subjective world of the person with dementia as its starting point (Feil 1993). Kitwood recognised the centrality of understanding the individual needs of people with dementia to give a focus for interventions. He asserted very strongly that without empathy the care environment would remain cold (1997b). Stokes (2000) also highlights the understanding of subjective experience as key to working in a person-centred way with so-called challenging behaviour. Clare *et al.* define person-centred approaches to dementia care as focusing on individual experiences: '…understanding the experience of dementia in terms of the person's psychological responses and social context, and aiming to tailor help and support to match individual needs' (Clare *et al.* 2003, p.251).

In trying to understand the perspective of the person with dementia, we begin to see that we have more in common as people than we have differences.

How can we appreciate the perspective of someone with dementia?

Putting oneself in the shoes of someone with dementia is not an easy or trivial process. Can any of us really know what it is like to be another? The answer is no. There are ways, however, that can help us see things from the stand-point of another. Kitwood (1997c) described various ways by which dementia care practitioners could deepen their empathy toward people with dementia. These can be used in professional development and training. They include:

- listening to and reading direct accounts of the experience of those living with dementia

- attending carefully to the actions and words of people with dementia

- using imagination to understand the experience of dementia.

Direct accounts

It has only been relatively recently that the direct voices of people with dementia have been taken seriously. The title of Malcolm Goldsmith's book, *Hearing the Voice of People with Dementia* (Goldsmith 1996) has come to be used as a phrase that represents serious efforts to communicate at an emotional level. It used to be thought that, because of the symptoms of disorientation and dysphasia, people experiencing dementia could not communicate anything in a meaningful or reliable fashion.

Over recent years there has been a shift in focus. This is, in part, to do with the person-centred care movement itself. As people with dementia have stepped out from behind the disease label, the recognition that they have something important to say has grown. There is also a much greater acknowledgement that speaking directly on one's own behalf is deeply empowering. Also, people with dementia are being seen by specialists much earlier. It is much more difficult to dismiss what people have to say about their experience when they are early on in their dementia. This trend is part of a wider movement within mental health services in the UK that care providers need to work in partnership with service users.

Likewise, it has only really been in more recent years that researchers have written seriously about the perspective of individuals with dementia (e.g. Downs 1997; Gubrium 1989; Keady 1996). In dementia research, phenomenological research into the early experience of Alzheimer's (Clare 2002; Sabat 2001) is now well established. In quality of life research, self-report measures on subjective well-being (Brod *et al.* 1999) and satisfaction with care (Mozley *et al.* 1999) have been developed relatively recently. There is now a body of evidence that people with dementia can answer interview questions in a reliable manner and can be involved directly in the research process.

Similarly, in dementia care practice, engaging directly with people with dementia in a therapeutic sense is a relatively new phenomenon (Bender and Cheston 1997). Personal accounts of living with dementia are very powerful as the quotations from Christine Bryden used in this book illustrate. The UK Alzheimer's Society's 'Living with Dementia' project and the views of people with dementia worldwide via www.dasninternational.org (DASN International) is a ready way in which we can access part of the experience of what it might be like to experience dementia.

Attending carefully

As verbal communication becomes more difficult, attending carefully to the non-verbal behaviour or piecing together fragmented speech becomes increasingly important. The work of John Killick and Kate Allan (Killick and Allan 2001) has been extremely influential in the UK in helping practitioners attend to the person with dementia in imaginative, creative and reflective ways. Killick and Allan (2006) describe their work with people with advanced dementia who are near to death, based on 'coma work' principles and using video and sound recordings paying very close attention to detail:

> We have no sense of time passing, so we live in the present reality, with no past and no future. We put all of our energy into now, not then or later. Sometimes this causes us a lot of anxiety because we worry about the past or the future because we cannot 'feel' that it exists. But this fact that we live in the present, with a depth of spirit and some tangled emotions, rather than cognition, means you can connect with us at a deep level through touch, eye contact, smiles. (Bryden 2005, p.99)

Another way of helping people to attend more carefully is through training them in a structured observation technique. Dementia Care Mapping (DCM) is, in part, an attempt to help care practitioners attend and observe with great care. Kitwood defined DCM thus: 'DCM is a serious attempt to take the standpoint of the person with dementia, using a combination of empathy and observational skill' (Kitwood 1997a, p.4).

A number of practitioners have written about the impact of observing this way, which reveals to them aspects of people's lives that they would never have noticed in their day-to-day work. Vera Bidder, a nursing assistant (Packer 1996), described how DCM changed her empathic response to people with dementia in her care:

> Shortly after the (DCM) course I became very conscious of the detractions that were still going on...I was bathing a person who was having difficulty forming a conversation. The door was flung open and the curtain pulled back. I protested, and the response was 'It's only a patient!' I was livid because it felt like it was me. I was the person having their privacy invaded. I found myself apologising to the person involved even though it wasn't my fault. (p.22)

Although DCM is a way of formally observing care in the communal areas of care settings, it is evident from the feedback we receive following training courses that teaching care workers to attend more carefully to the perspective of people with dementia greatly deepens their level of empathy across all care situations.

DCM provides care teams with feedback about how the people in their care are experiencing daily life. Through such a process, staff are empowered to consider care from the point of view of the person with dementia (Brooker, Edwards and Benson 2004).

Using the imagination

Using the imagination to put oneself in the place of someone trying to cope with the symptoms of dementia is a very powerful means of increasing empathy. The symptoms of disorientation, dysphasias and dyspraxias are often described but it is how these make people feel that is often overlooked.

Working in the field of dementia care, you learn very quickly that the emotional reactions that people with dementia experience are as strong as they ever were. Although there is a decline in cognitive abilities, there is no decline in depth of feeling. Indeed for many people, emotions appear stronger than ever, partly because of the decline in the volitional control of emotions that can be part and parcel of dementia. Anger, joy, grief and excitement are often easily accessed.

In conversation with people with dementia, there is a constant interplay between memories that are well stored and what is going on in the here and now. Past events and memories feel much more present than recent ones. Present events will trigger past memories. What is happening in the present moment has a significant impact on how the person feels. In person-centred training sessions, I often ask staff to do a guided fantasy exercise using their own memories and personalities in interplay with some of the symptoms common in dementia. An example of this is described in the box below.

A DCM trainer explains a guided fantasy exercise to deepen empathy

I ask the staff team to imagine themselves a little older than now sitting in a dementia care setting they know well. I get them to picture exactly where they are sitting, what they can see from that position, what the people look like. Who passes by? What do they look like? What are they wearing? What noises can they hear? What smells can they smell? I describe that they do not know this place but it seems sort of familiar. They have no idea how they got there or how to get home. They can't think where the car is and they have no money, credit cards or keys. They have a bad feeling about some of the people around them and good feelings about some of the others. They think they might know a couple of the people but can't for the life of them remember any of their names. Other people seem to know their name; others call them by a name they don't recognise.

I describe symptoms of communication difficulties – that they find it very difficult to explain what they want and frequently lose the thread of conversation and cannot find the right word. I explain that their movements feel clumsy and even simple tasks that they know they should be able to do, elude them. I explain that maybe they have a pain but they do not know why. I describe how their emotions are still the same. What makes them smile and laugh still makes them smile and laugh and the things that make them want to cry, still make them want to cry.

At the end of the exercise I ask them what it is they want? What could help alleviate some of their distress? On the other hand I ask what they wouldn't want to happen to them? What might add to their distress? Using their own long-term memories, I ask them to imagine where they think they are. I also ask as an observer, what I would see them doing.

At the end of this exercise the specific things that people want vary according to their personal histories and personalities. The vast majority of people want gentle and kind human contact. Many wish to be held, a few do not. All wish that someone would take their fears seriously. All wish that someone would take the time to reach out to them, for many feel disempowered to do this for themselves. None want to be ignored, patronised, brushed off or rushed. People imagine they are in all kinds of places but school, work and 'definitely not at home' are common responses. Behaviours that many describe are to escape or to search for something comforting and familiar. Others claim that they would become quite aggressive, particularly if they were prevented from leaving. The majority claim that they would sit quietly, tense and vigilant, hoping that no-one would hurt them. (Brooker and Surr 2005, p.20)

This sort of exercise can be very powerful. It increases empathy and awareness of the needs of others. It decreases the distance between 'us' and 'them'. It helps us to recognise that we are all human and dependent on each other for our survival.

Role play and other methods that engage poetic imagination are sometimes routes to epiphanic knowledge (Hawkins 2005) – the understanding achieved in flashes of insight, so-called 'light bulb' moments when the penny drops or the scales fall from our eyes. Film, poetry, fiction, personal accounts and observations, or conversations with clients can all be a route to epiphanic knowledge.

In DCM, trainers use role play to deepen their empathy of the lived experience of dementia as well as using it to help trainees observe accurately. Even with this group of people who will already have considered the lived experience of people with dementia, role play can be a route to epiphanic knowledge. I remember working with a very experienced dementia care practitioner who was training to be a DCM trainer but who was very anxious about role play. His anxiety centred on giving a perfect performance in demonstrating the codes. He decided to base it on a patient that he knew well so that he could get the mannerisms just right. One of the behaviours that he had to demonstrate was calling out in a distressed manner and receiving no response. He confided to me afterwards that it had been a very odd experience and he had found himself calling out for his wife – something that he had no intention of doing. This provided him with direct knowledge about attachment needs in people with dementia that he had previously only understood at an intellectual level.

Personal perspectives in practice

What follows are a series of questions to help your organisation reflect on where you are in terms of the Personal Perspectives element of person-centred care.

The indicators in the Personal Perspectives element of VIPS primarily need to be led by those who are responsible for the day-to-day management of direct care staff and the direct service environment. These indicators are about the way in which direct care staff respond to their caring role and how they demonstrate empathy with those they care for.

Having responsibility for the direct operational management of a service or leading shifts within a service is a tough job. It often feels as if everyone comes to you with their problems. Balancing the needs of an over-worked staff group, covering shifts, dealing with sickness, new admissions, deaths and illness, worried relatives, angry relatives and having to attend meetings that go on for hours are all in a day's work for people in this position. All this can easily take precedence over being a role model for staff and ensuring that their day-to-day interactions are of a high standard. If no one is complaining, then it is easy to think that there is no problem.

Providing person-centred care that really takes the perspective of people with dementia – particularly those with more advanced dementia – is a tough challenge. Complaints about this area are not common – unless there is a high level of challenging behaviour in which case the expectation will be that you need to 'sort it' out or 'manage it'. The fact that you are reading this chapter means that you take this endeavour seriously and have a desire to be proactive in ensuring that the people you care for get the best possible opportunity for having their needs understood.

What follows is a series of questions to help care providers benchmark where they are in terms of the Personal Perspective element of person-centred care. These questions will help care providers explore how well they try to look at life from the perspective of the person with dementia using their services.

---

1. Communication with service users

On a day-to-day basis, are service users asked for their preferences, consent and opinions?

In order to know a person's opinion, it is important that they are asked directly about this! It is surprising how often, however, this basic courtesy and social interaction does not occur in services for people with dementia. This occurs for a number of reasons. The first is the belief that the person with dementia cannot make a reliable comment, and the second is that it will take too long to do. Although people may lose the capacity to make truly informed choices about abstract decisions as time goes by, the evidence is that people can make reliable decisions about long-held preferences well into their dementia. Even if the capacity for understanding language is severely impaired, the non-verbal behaviour that accompanies being asked for permission or opinion will not go unnoticed and will do much to convey to the person with dementia that they are worth bothering about.

This is different from user involvement activities where people may be interviewed or surveyed about their views. What I am describing here is the everyday practice of asking for people's opinions on what they want to eat or drink, where they would like to sit and what they need to feel comfortable. On a day-to-day basis, are attempts made to discuss these sorts of issues directly with the person with dementia? Are the direct care staff good communicators generally? Do they recognise the barriers to communication due to sensory disability and have strategies to overcome these? Do they recognise the barriers to communication due to cognitive disabilities and have strategies to overcome these?

When decisions need to be made that are either too complex or abstract for the service user with dementia to make an informed decision about, do staff talk to people who know them well, such as family, and who can often offer insight into their past preferences?

Is this backed up by observations of the person in different situations to attempt or confirm a best estimation of their wishes?

This can be evidenced by direct observation of practice. In a DCM evaluation, this would be evidenced by a high occurrence of Personal Enhancers such as negotiation, collaboration, enabling and respect in environments where communication is high on the agenda. There would also be evidence of a higher level of engagement overall, particularly with staff.

Knowing the opinion, wishes and goals of the service user should also be apparent from an audit of assessment processes and care plans. Is the perspective of the service user represented within all paperwork relating to them?

---

2. Empathy and acceptable risk

Do staff show the ability to put themselves in the position of the person they are caring for and to think about decisions from their point of view?

There will be occasions and decisions where the person with dementia is unable to fully participate and put forward their own point of view. It is important then that staff are able to try to think things through from the viewpoint of the person with dementia. This may be particularly important around issues of risk assessment.

There is often tremendous pressure to err on the side of caution with regards to situations that may include an element of risk. People with dementia are a vulnerable group within our society and it is wholly right that those responsible for their care work to ensure their safety. People with dementia are, however, in danger of being kept so safe that they have no quality of life at all. Because of memory problems and impaired communication abilities, people with dementia often cannot express their wishes and it is easy to err so much on the side of safety that life becomes little more than eating, sleeping and toileting.

There are hidden dangers and risks that exist to emotional well-being in the form of boredom, helplessness, depression and giving up. Often, it will be up to the person's key worker or a professional to advocate on behalf of their emotional well-being. Being able to use information about what the person enjoys doing now and what their past interests were (see Chapter 3) will help inform choices.

In order to put this into practice, are staff able to tell if a person with dementia is in a state of relative well-being or ill-being? Can they identify, describe and respond appropriately to verbal and non-verbal signs of well- and ill-being? Is this done as part of a decision-making process about risk?

In auditing risk assessment documentation and care plans, it is useful to see whether decisions have been made purely on the basis of physical safety, or whether attempts have been made to look at various options and activities from the point of view of the service user and their emotional well-being. In observation of practice, the Personal Enhancers of relaxed pace, validation and facilitation, present alongside low levels of withdrawn and distressed states, would also indicate that staff are working at an empathic level.

---

3. Physical environment

Is the physical environment – e.g. noise, temperature – managed on a day-to-day basis to help people with dementia feel at ease?

People with dementia are often at the mercy of other people controlling their physical environment. Imagine being in your 80s, living with a dementia, confined to a chair because you can no longer manage to walk, sitting for ten hours a day in the same lounge in the same chair in the same position. The radio in the next lounge is constantly tuned to pop music; the TV in your lounge alternates between soap operas and children's pro-grammes set at a constantly high volume; you cannot see out of any of the windows because the sills are above your eye line; a loud call bell goes off at unpredictable intervals; a different bell goes off every time someone leaves or enters the front door; footsteps echo down the uncarpeted corridors; the hearing aid of the person sitting next to you whistles all day; and you are cold. This is the reality of the lived experience of many people living in care homes. Attention may have been paid to the physi-cal design of such facilities – they may even have won architec-tural awards – but, unless the micro-environment is managed so that people are comfortable, then such endeavour is worthless.

On a day-to-day basis, it is important that staff use their empathic skills to be actively aware of the comfort needs of people with dementia. Often people with dementia may not be able to tell staff directly that they are in discomfort or they may not be able to work out for themselves how to alleviate discom-fort. This may occur many times over the course of a day.

Let's consider a few such incidences that might occur in the morning. At breakfast, a cup placed too far away may get ignored and the person will not drink and remain thirsty; while getting dressed, a garment may be put on incorrectly causing skin to become sore; sitting in a chair by the window in the sun may cause the person to become too hot, and the glare of the sun into the room may mean they do not see the drinks trolley coming round. The thirst continues. The person becomes anxious and begins to pace about trying to find a way to stop the discom-fort. None of these incidents on its own is major but, if allowed to continue, their cumulative effect can be devastating, even leading to some of the challenging behaviours outlined later.

Incidents such as these are often picked up by direct obser-vation of practice such as DCM. In busy care environments, it is easy for this sort of scenario to unfold unless steps are taken to minimise the risk of this happening. Where the staff group is highly empathic, during a DCM evaluation this would be evi-denced by a high occurrence of Personal Enhancers such as warmth, holding, relaxed pace, validation and facilitation. One of the insights most often gained through a DCM evaluation is into the level of distress caused by environmental factors that are easily remediable once they have been noted as problematic.

An awareness of the micro-environment of a sitting room can only be experienced through sitting in a place for a good length of time. A period sitting and soaking up the atmosphere in one of the lounges can be most enlightening. What might feel like a busy and productive workplace can feel very differently when you experience the service from the point of view of a service user. Is there a welcoming ambiance? Are temperature and noise levels acceptable, and is there a balance of sensory rich areas with quiet space?

---

4. Physical health

Are the physical health needs of people with dementia including pain assessment, sight and hearing problems, given due attention?

As we saw in Chapter 2, people with dementia are prone to having physical health problems that can go undetected for a long time if staff around them are not vigilant about investigating causes of any sudden increase in confusion. When caring for a person with dementia, any sudden increase in the level of confusion should be treated with the suspicion that there could be a physical health problem contributing to the general confusion. Physical fitness and comfort need to be taken seriously. Poor physical health greatly intensifies the impairments caused by dementia. Pain is often undetected in people with dementia, and the manifestations of the person's discomfort may be misperceived as episodes of 'challenging behaviour'. As people with dementia may have difficulty remembering episodes of pain or difficulty finding the words to describe their symptoms, the onus has to be on the carers to be proactive in this respect.

Unaddressed age-related sensory impairments such as not having the correct spectacles or functioning hearing aids often lie at the root of communication problems. If someone has poor visual perception and dysphasia due to their dementia, this only gets worse if they do not have all the help they can get from physical prostheses. Again, because of their dementia, an individual may not be able to say that they have lost their glasses or to complain that their hearing aid no longer functions. Professionals and care staff have to be vigilant on their behalf.

Again, this can be evidenced through an audit of care plans, particularly with reference to pain management. An analysis of hospital admissions will sometimes show up whether or not physical health problems are being picked up too late. An audit of glasses, hearing aids and dentures may also be illuminating.

---

5. Challenging behaviour as communication

Is 'challenging behaviour' analysed to discover the underlying reasons for it?

A great deal has been written about the need to understand so-called challenging behaviour from the perspective of the person with dementia.

This term covers a number of behaviours but particularly here I would include heightened distress, aggression, anxiety, paranoia, inappropriate sexual behaviour, low mood, withdrawal and self-harm.

As Christine Bryden writes:

The world goes much faster than we do, whizzing around, and we are being asked to do things, or to respond, or to play a game, or to participate in group activities. It is too fast, we want to say 'Go away, slow down, leave me alone, just go away' and maybe we might then be difficult, not co-operative. Challenging behaviour? I believe that this is 'adaptive behaviour', where I am adapting to my care environment. (Bryden 2005, p128)

In person-centred care, we try to see meaning in all behaviour and use this as a starting point for trying to help those in distress. The first step is in trying to understand the function of the be-haviour for the individual and what the person is trying to tell us by the behaviour. This is particularly evident when people with dementia are in distress but cannot explain this through normal channels. Thus we might see the person act in a way that has been labelled as challenging behaviour such as verbal or physi-cal aggression, self-harm, shouting out, repetitive questioning, escape behaviours, paranoid behaviours, accusatory behaviours, socially inappropriate behaviours and sexually inappropriate be-haviours. These are very distressing behaviours both to the person experiencing them and to those in a caring role.

A person-centred response would be to see the challenge in them as one that challenges us as a care team to find the reasons underlying the behaviour and to help the person achieve a state of well-being. In understanding the perspective of the service user and using this as part of our detailed analysis, we can then have a plan that supports personhood.

The reasons underlying challenging behaviours can usually be understood by reference to the Enriched Model of dementia. Is there something about this person's cognitive disability that means they are misinterpreting or becoming overwhelmed by their situation? Is there something in their past life that is being triggered by their current situation that is causing distress? Is there a mismatch between their preferences and needs and what the current environment is offering? Is there an untreated physical complaint that is causing an increase in confusion or pain? Is the level of social care meeting their personhood needs?

The practice of being proactive, and to always consider what a situation may look and feel like to the person with dementia, should lead to a lower incidence of challenging behaviour. I have worked on many challenging behaviour units in my time which are characterised by an atmosphere of relative calm. To the casual visitor, it will look as if staff are doing very little apart from spending time with people as needed. This belies the fact that the team will have spent time learning all about the viewpoint of those they are caring for and putting it into everyday practice. The problem with these units is when people are transferred to facilities where staff do not have the skills. The challenging behaviour re-occurs very quickly if people are placed back in situations where staff do not have the ability to try to put themselves in the position of the person for whom they are caring.

A non-person-centred response sees challenging behaviour primarily as part and parcel of the dementia that cannot be helped but has to be managed. The response in this case would be restraint, behavioural management and medication – or a combination of all three.

Finding out whether this occurs in practice can be shown by a care plan audit to see whether reasons have been sought for challenging behaviours. Often a look at the level of prescribing of neuroleptic medication will indicate whether this is a first-line response to challenging behaviour or not.

---

6. Advocacy

In situations where the actions of an individual with dementia are at odds with the safety and well-being of others, how are the rights of the individual protected?

The most difficult situations that staff and residents face in long-term care settings are when the rights of one individual are at odds with the safety and comfort of others. An example of this might arise within a housing facility where a resident who is disorientated is constantly knocking on neighbours' doors. Another example could be within a residential home where a resident has become sexually disinhibited and is making sexual advances to others that are not welcomed. In such a situation, the initial response is that the person who is causing the problem should be removed to another facility. The problem with this response is that it may actually exacerbate the problem for the individual concerned and simply make it someone else's responsibility. In some cases, it may truly be the case that the individual's needs can be met better elsewhere because of better trained staff or higher staffing ratios.

There is no simple solution to situations such as these, but they occur with enough regularity that some mechanism for dealing with them needs to be in place before they occur. This sort of situation usually gives rise to a case conference or case review, and the person who may not be able to argue their own corner should have someone advocating on their behalf. In some situations, this might be a social worker or a community nurse. In other situations, it might be that the organisation calls on the services of a formal advocacy service.

How a care provider deals with these situations can be evidenced by a review of policies and procedures and also looking at the circumstances surrounding people being moved on.

Summary

Element Three of person-centred care is about providing care that tries to look at life from the perspective of the service user. Care is provided in a way where the priority is placed on promoting the well-being of people with dementia. The degree to which organisations take the viewpoint of people with dementia seriously can be seen in reactions to and levels of so-called challenging behaviour, day-to-day communication, empathic ability of care staff, vigilance around physical health and advocacy services.

5

Social Environment

**Element Four of person centred-care
is providing a social environment that
supports psychological needs**

Providing a supportive social environment: recognising
that all human life is grounded in relationships and that
people with dementia need an enriched social
environment which both compensates for their
impairment and fosters opportunities for personal
growth.

Key indicators for care providers on the social environment

- **INCLUSION:** Are people with dementia helped by
  staff to be included in conversations and helped to
  relate to others? Is there an absence of people being
  'talked across'?

- **RESPECT:** Are all service users treated with respect with an absence of people being demeaned by 'tellings off' or labelling?

- **WARMTH:** Is there an atmosphere of warmth and acceptance to service users? Do people look comfortable or intimidated and neglected?

- **VALIDATION:** Are people's fears taken seriously? Are people left alone for long periods in emotional distress?

- **ENABLING:** Do staff help people with dementia to be active in their own care and activity? Is there an absence of people being treated like objects with no feelings?

- **PART OF THE COMMUNITY:** Is there evidence of service users using local community facilities and people from the local community visiting regularly?

How you relate to us has a big impact on the course of the disease. You can restore our personhood, and give us a sense of being needed and valued. There is a Zulu saying that is very true. 'A person is a person through others.' Give us reassurance, hugs, support, a meaning in life. Value us for what we can still do and be, and make sure we retain social networks. It is very hard for us to be who we once were, so let us be who we are now and realise the effort we are making to function. (Bryden 2005, p.127)

In providing person-centred care, a supportive and nurturing social environment is the key to maintaining personhood on a day-to-day basis. Personhood can only be maintained in the context of relationships. Carl Rogers saw relationships as key to therapeutic growth and change. He highlighted the importance of the relationship and therapeutic alliance in person-centred counselling. Kitwood's view of person-centred care for people with dementia was that it took place in the context of relationships – *Person to Person* was the title of Kitwood and Bredin's 1992c publication which was the first book on person-centred dementia care in practice. With the onset of dementia individuals are very vulnerable to their psychological defences being broken down. As the sense of self breaks down, it becomes increasingly important that the sense of self is held within the relationships that the person with dementia experiences. John Bond also includes the context of relationships within his description of personhood: '…individuals do not function in isolation, they also have relationships with others; all human life is interconnected and interdependent' (Bond 2001, p.47).

The maintenance of relationships is not dependent on verbal skills. As Ian Morton (1999) points out, as verbal abilities are lost, the importance of warm, accepting human contact through non-verbal channels becomes even more important. Also, people with dementia may be more aware of any incongruence in what is being communicated verbally and non-verbally, because of their stronger reliance on non-verbal communication.

Sabat's (2001) demonstration of social positioning with respect to people with dementia lends empirical support to the manner in which interactions enhance or diminish a person's sense of self. His work also provides evidence of the way people with dementia actively cope with how they are treated.

The importance of conceptualising the person with dementia in relationship to others has been underlined by the coining of the term 'relationship-centred care'. Mike Nolan (Nolan, Davies and Grant 2001) offers a very useful framework about conceptualising relationships in care homes based on developing a sense of security, continuity, belonging, purpose, achievement and significance. This is well articulated in the in-depth report *My Home Life* (Help the Aged 2006).

Malignant Social Psychology and Positive Person Work

As with all the elements of person-centred care, ensuring that people with dementia have the opportunity for social and loving relationships with those around them seems so obvious that surely we do not need a set of guidelines to achieve this? However, again even a cursory examination of care provision shows that this is not the norm in care practice. Kitwood's writing on Malignant Social Psychology (MSP) helps to clarify why this seems so difficult to achieve in practice.

Kitwood (1997a) described personhood being undermined by an MSP of care where people with dementia experience dehumanising interactions which include being stigmatised, invalidated and ignored. This Malignant Social Psychology is rarely created with any malicious intent; rather, it becomes woven into the culture of care. The impact of this on the well-being of people with dementia, who are already struggling to adapt to neurological impairment and to maintain their sense of self, is hypothesised as being psychologically damaging.

Concrete examples of MSP are provided in the description of 17 types of Personal Detractions in Dementia Care Mapping (DCM). Descriptions of the 17 types of Personal Detractions (MSP) alongside an example of each are now presented.[1] In these examples, George, Lorna, Frank and Elizabeth are all residents with dementia living in a care home. The examples all centre on a meal time. Although these are hypothetical examples, they are similar to the ones DCM evaluators have noted as part of routine care.

1   All these examples of Personal Detractions were produced by my colleague Hazel May.

1. **INTIMIDATION:** Making a participant frightened
    or fearful by using spoken threats or physical power.

    George is sitting at the dining table; he has eaten a
    few mouthfuls of main course but has now put his
    fork down. A care worker walks past and says to him,
    'George, if you don't eat up I'll tell your wife and
    she'll be really cross with you.'

2. **WITHHOLDING:** Refusing to give asked-for
    attention, or to meet an evident need for contact.

    It is hectic in the lounge. Staff are busily helping
    people to move from the sitting room to the dining
    area. Lorna is still in her chair and reaches out for
    contact with a passing staff member; the staff
    member dodges out of her way and carries on
    towards the dining area.

3. **OUTPACING:** Providing information and
    presenting choices at a rate too fast for a participant
    to understand.

    Elizabeth is being fed by a member of staff who taps
    her lower lip with the spoon in between mouthfuls to
    prompt her to eat more quickly.

4. **INFANTILISATION:** Treating a participant in a
    patronising way as if she or he were a small child.

    At the end of the meal, the care worker says, 'There's
    a good girl,' to Elizabeth.

5. **LABELLING:** Using a label as the main way to
    describe or relate to a participant.

    Lorna is still in the lounge. One of the care workers
    asks the nurse in charge if she should feed her. The
    nurse replies, 'Leave her till the end, she's one of the
    screachers.'

6. **DISPARAGEMENT:** Telling a participant that he or she is incompetent, useless, worthless, incapable.

George is still sitting at the dining table with his half eaten meal. 'Come on George this is no good at all, you can do better than this,' says one of the care workers.

7. **ACCUSATION:** Blaming a participant for things they have done, or have not been able to do.

Frank has been waiting at the table for his meal to arrive. He is sitting next to George who has not touched his food for some time. Frank pulls George's meal in front of him and starts to eat it. A care worker quickly comes over and tells him off: 'That's not your food Frank and you know it.'

8. **TREACHERY:** Using trickery or deception to distract or manipulate a participant in order to make them do or not do something.

The care worker then tries to help George to finish his dinner. She tells him, 'Come on George, just eat a few more mouthfuls, then I'll phone your wife and tell her how good you've been.'

9. **INVALIDATION:** Failing to acknowledge the reality of a participant in a particular situation.

George tells her he's not hungry; she replies, 'That can't be true George, it's dinner time and you always eat your dinner.'

10. **DISEMPOWERMENT:** Not allowing a participant to use the abilities that they do have.

Elizabeth tries to hold on to the spoon that the care worker is feeding her with. The care worker gently moves Elizabeth's hand away and guides it to her lap where she keeps hold of it to stop her repeating the attempt.

11. **IMPOSITION:** Forcing a participant to do something, over-riding their own desires or wishes, or denying them choice.

Lunch time is over. Frank has finished drinking his tea but is holding on to the mug. A member of the domestic staff who is clearing the tables tries to take the mug from him. He holds on tight so she peels his fingers away from the mug one at a time and takes it away.

12. **DISRUPTION:** Intruding on or interfering with something a participant is doing, or crudely breaking her or his 'frame of reference'.

Lorna has dozed off and now one of the care workers wants to give her lunch. The care worker gives Lorna a little gentle shake and tells her its lunch time. Lorna looks groggy and disorientated as the care worker pulls her to her feet.

13. **OBJECTIFICATION:** Treating a participant as if he or she were a lump of dead matter or an object.

A care worker comes up behind George and reverses his wheelchair away from the table before proceeding to wheel him into the lounge.

14. **STIGMATISATION:** Treating a participant as if they were a diseased object, alien or outcast.

Lorna is being helped into the lounge for a late dinner on her own. 'Sit her over there where she can't bother other people,' says the domestic to the care worker.

15. **IGNORING:** Carrying on (in conversation or action) in the presence of a participant as if he or she is not there.

    'Actually, she's not been too bad today,' comes the reply.

16. **BANISHMENT:** Sending a participant away, or excluding her or him, physically or psychologically.

    Frank wanders back into the dining room and is told, 'You're not allowed in here now Frank, go back to the lounge please.'

17. **MOCKERY:** Making fun of a participant; teasing, humiliating them and making jokes at their expense.

    The domestic and the care worker in the dining room laugh at Frank as he walks away; his trousers are gradually slipping down.

Kitwood was at pains to say that episodes of MSP are very rarely done with any malicious intent. Rather, episodes of MSP become interwoven into the care culture. This way of responding to people in care gets learnt in the same way that new staff learn to fold sheets. If you are a new staff member in a nursing home, you learn how to communicate with residents from other staff with whom you work. If their communication style with residents is one that is characterised by infantilisation and outpacing, then you will follow their lead. The malignancy in MSP is that it eats away at the personhood of those being cared for, and also it spreads from one member of staff to another very quickly.

In a DCM evaluation, all episodes of Personal Detractions that are observed are recorded and fed back to the care team. Once care teams become consciously aware of episodes of Personal Detractions and tackle them as part of a practice development process, the incidence of them often radically decreases.

Kitwood also described what a positive social psychology might look like for people with dementia. If personhood is undermined by MSP then it should also be possible to describe the sorts of everyday interactions that would promote the maintenance of personhood. He used the term 'Positive Person Work' to describe ten different forms of interaction that would maintain personhood. These were labelled recognition, negotiation, collaboration, play, timalation (engagement through the senses), celebration, relaxation, validation, holding and facilitation (1997a, pp.90–3).

In the development of DCM 8, an expanded list of descriptions of Personal Enhancers that would enhance well-being and maintain personhood was developed. Positive Person Work was used as a starting point in the development of Personal Enhancers. Personal Enhancers are not intended to be the polar opposite of Personal Detractions. Rather, they describe an alternative way of interacting.

In the following examples, George, Lorna, Frank and Elizabeth have a much better experience over their lunch time. Again, although these are hypothetical examples, they are similar to the ones DCM evaluators have noted as part of care practice.[2]

1. **WARMTH:** Demonstrating genuine affection, care and concern for the participant.

    George is in the dining room; he has only eaten a small amount of his dinner. A care worker comes and sits with him. She asks him if he is feeling unwell, or if there is anything she can do to help him enjoy his dinner. George explains that he isn't feeling too good today; the care worker tells him she is sorry to hear this; she asks if he would rather have just a cup of tea and some toast, to which he replies, 'Yes please.'

---

2   All the examples of Personal Enhancers were produced by my colleague Hazel May.

2. **HOLDING:** Providing safety, security and comfort to a participant.

It is lunch time and the lounge is hectic and noisy. Lorna begins to become distressed and starts to scream. A care worker comes to her and makes eye contact, holds her hand and gently talks to her explaining that it is lunch time and that people are moving into the dining room. She stays with her until things have calmed down and then asks her if she would like some food.

3. **RELAXED PACE:** Recognising the importance of helping to create a relaxed atmosphere.

A care worker is helping Elizabeth with her meal. He is at eye level with Elizabeth explaining what is on the spoon and letting Elizabeth set the pace. He waits for Elizabeth to finish each mouthful and waits for her to open her mouth before giving her more.

4. **RESPECT:** Treating the participant as a valued member of society and recognising their experience and age.

Lorna has come into the dining room and is looking anxious; she picks up a table mat and starts to walk away with it. A care worker walks alongside and thanks her for being patient about the delay of her meal. She asks her whether she would like to take the place mat into the lounge and eat on her own or to return to the dining room.

5. **ACCEPTANCE:** Entering into a relationship based on an attitude of acceptance or positive regard for the participant.

Frank has started to eat George's dinner. A care worker asks him if he would like a fresher, hotter serving of food than the one he has, to which he replies, 'No thank you.' The care worker then offers George a fresh, hot serving to which the he replies, 'No thanks, I've had enough.'

6. **CELEBRATION:** Recognising, supporting and taking delight in the skills and achievements of the participant.

Dinner time is over but Frank is still holding on to his empty cup. A member of staff who is clearing up congratulates him on always eating and enjoying his food so much. 'It makes my job a pleasure,' she says to him and then asks him if he'd like his mug refilling.

7. **ACKNOWLEDGEMENT:** Recognising, accepting and supporting the participant as unique, and valuing them as an individual.

Lorna has indicated that she would rather eat alone in the lounge. The care worker finds a coffee table for her and helps Lorna to put the place mat on the table. 'I know how you feel,' says the care worker, 'it's so noisy in there and you've always been more comfortable away from crowds, haven't you Lorna, and that's just fine, don't worry.'

8. **GENUINENESS:** Being honest and open with the participant in a way that is sensitive to their needs and feelings.

As Lorna finishes her dinner she says she would like to go home now. The care worker says, 'Do you feel tired Lorna, do you want to go home so that you can lie down?' 'Yes,' replies Lorna. 'Well, I know this isn't your home but you do have a room with a nice comfy bed here and we could go there now so that you can have a rest, would that do?'

9. **VALIDATION:** Recognising and supporting the reality of the participant. Sensitivity to feeling and emotion take priority.

Lorna says that she needs her mother. The care worker replies, 'Yes, I know what you mean, are you feeling a bit lost at the moment? I know I'm not your mother but is there anything I could do for you?'

10. **EMPOWERMENT:** Letting go of control and assisting the participant to discover or employ abilities and skills.

Elizabeth tries to take hold of the spoon as she is being fed. The care worker guides Elizabeth's hand to the spoon and helps her to hold it; they both hold the spoon and guide it together.

11. **FACILITATION:** Assessing the level of support required and providing it.

The care worker lets go of Elizabeth's hand to see if she can manage alone, but quickly resumes his support when Elizabeth nearly drops the spoon.

12. **ENABLING:** Recognising and encouraging a participant's level of engagement within a frame of reference.

George is still sitting in his wheelchair at the table and starts to propel himself backwards and forwards. A care worker asks him if he would like to move away from the table. 'Yes,' comes the reply. The care worker helps George to reverse away from the table and then asks him if he would like to push himself towards the lounge – George is delighted and starts his journey back to the lounge.

13. **COLLABORATION:** Treating the participant as a full and equal partner in what is happening, consulting and working with them.

Lorna has said that she would like to go and lie down now. The care worker helps Lorna step-by-step to get up from her chair, to walk across the lounge and to find her bedroom. At each stage, she explains what is happening and offers Lorna the opportunity to make her own decisions.

14. **RECOGNITION:** Meeting the participant in his or her own uniqueness, bringing an open and unprejudiced attitude.

Elizabeth has finished eating and gets cross with the care worker who has been feeding her; she scowls at him. The care worker says, 'Don't worry Elizabeth, I haven't forgotten that you always have a cup of sweet tea after your meal, I'll go and get it for you now.'

15. **INCLUDING:** Enabling and encouraging the participant to be and feel included, physically and psychologically.

Frank goes back into the dining room while the domestic staff are clearing up. One of them says to him, 'Hello Frank, nice to see you, come and give us a hand if you like.'

16. **BELONGING:** Providing a sense of acceptance in a particular setting regardless of abilities and disabilities.

George arrives back in the lounge after his meal. A member of staff greets him, 'Hello George, I've been waiting for you, here's your newspaper, I know you like a rest and a read after lunch, and I was hoping I could join you.'

17. **FUN:** Accessing a free, creative way of being and using and responding to the use of fun and humour.

Frank has joined in helping some of the staff to clear the tables after lunch. Staff make sure he is included in the jokes and banter and he laughs and jokes in the group.

In a DCM evaluation, all examples of Personal Enhancers are described and fed back to the care team. Again, through a process of practice development, this reinforces person-centred interactions and increases the likelihood of their becoming the norm. It is not necessary to be DCM-trained to recognise Personal Detractions or Personal Enhancers. They appear to be familiar aspects of care around the world. Jane Verity and Dan Kuhn (Verity and Kuhn, in press) offer many further descriptions based on Personal Detractions and alternative ways of responding, called Put-downs and Up-lifts.

Psychological needs

MSP and Positive Person Work relate directly to the psychological needs that Kitwood identified. Kitwood wrote and talked about what people with dementia needed from those around them to enable them to exist as a person. He chose a flower with overlapping petals to illustrate these needs, with love being the central need in the heart of the flower. This is the type of unconditional acceptance that is generous and forgiving and asks for no reward. If we truly love another, we will seek unstintingly to provide what they need to thrive.

There are many care workers who have the ability to love the people they care for in this way. It does not need to be taught to them. Indeed, sometimes in our rush to become professional or expert, that initial motivation of love for people we care for can get lost along the way.

As we become more emotional and less cognitive, it's the way you talk to us, not what you say, that we will remember. We know the feeling, but don't know the plot. Your smile, your laugh and your touch are what we will connect with. Empathy heals. Just love us as we are. We're still here, in emotion and spirit, if only you could find us. (Bryden 2005, p.138)

For others this type of love for those we care for does not come naturally. By looking at the needs that people have in turn, however, most of us can recognise ways by which we can meet those needs and help to maintain personhood.

Comfort

This is the provision of warmth and closeness to others. Comfort is about the provision of tenderness, closeness and soothing. It promotes security and decreases anxiety. It helps people relax. Comfort can be provided through physical touch, or through comforting words or gestures. Comfort also includes physical comfort with one's body. A lack of comfort will be experienced by those who are in pain, or who feel physically ill or unwell, or who are sitting or lying in an unpleasant place.

My stress tolerance is very low, and even a minor disruption can cause a catastrophic reaction, where I shout or scream, panic and pace. I need calm, no surprises, no sudden changes. Anxiety is an undercurrent of our disease. I feel I have to do something but can't remember what and often it feels like something terrible is going to happen, but I have forgotten what it is. With the stress of many activities at once, I become very focused, trying with all the brain I have left to concentrate. Telling me to rest won't help, but helping me to complete the task will. (Bryden 2005 p.111)

Identity

This relates to the need to know who you are and how you feel about yourself and how you think. Often, as the recent memories fade and language becomes problematic, identity is increasingly provided by those around the person with dementia. Identity relates to knowing who one is and to having a sense of continuity with the past. It is also about having a life story that is held and maintained, either by the person with dementia, or for them by others. Others know about you, they know who you are and they hold you in esteem. Identity can be undermined particularly by infantilisation, labelling and disparagement. Identity is supported by respect, acceptance and celebrations.

> Please don't call us 'dementing' – we are still people separate from our disease, we just have a disease of the brain. If I had cancer you would not refer to me as 'cancerous' would you? (Bryden 2005, p.143)

> Helen said she often felt lost, even in her own home. It was not really a matter of losing her way, but losing herself somehow… Somehow in her head, there was no sense of being a person existing in this space. Helen said it was worse when she was by herself but when others related to her, she seemed to come back from somewhere where she had been lost. Maybe they acted like a mirror for her, reflecting her existence, reaffirming her personhood. (Bryden 2005, p.43)

Attachment

Human beings are a highly social species and need to feel attached to others particularly at times of heightened anxiety and change. Attachment relates to bonding, connection, nurture, trust and relationship. It also relates to security in relationships, and feeling that one has trusted others to whom one can turn in times of trouble or need. When people are anxious, the need to feel attached to someone or something familiar often increases to a significant degree. Attachment needs can be supported by acknowledgement, genuineness and validation. Attachment can be undermined by accusations, treachery and invalidation.

> The future looks bleak to the person with dementia – it not only looks bleak, but actually is bleak so I believe it is wrong to deny us help to deal with the whole gamut of emotions we will experience along the journey of this disease. (Bryden 2005, p.131)
>
> Try to enter our distorted reality, because if you make us fit in with your reality, it will cause us extra stress. (Bryden 2005, p.147)

Occupation

This relates to being involved in the process of life. It fulfils a deep need that individuals can have an impact on the world and those around them. Occupation relates to being involved in activity in a way that is personally meaningful. It also relates to having a sense of agency, which is about feeling one has control over the world and can make things happen. It is about feeling that you can have an effect and impact on what is done and how. Occupation is supported by empowering, enabling, facilitating and collaborative staff skills. Occupation is undermined by disempowerment, disruption, imposition and objectification.

We feel as if we are hanging onto a high cliff, above a lurking black hole. Daily tasks are complex. Nothing is automatic anymore. Everything is as if we are first learning. You tell us that we have asked you that question before, but we have no recollection. It is just a blank for the past and this feels strange and scary, and yet you are frustrated with us. If we had an arm or a leg missing you would congratulate us on our efforts but you cannot see how much of our brain is missing and how hard it is to cope so you don't understand our struggles. (Bryden 2005, p.98)

Inclusion

Being part of a group is important for the survival of the human species. People with dementia are at great risk of being socially isolated even when they live in a communal setting. If no effort is made to help people with dementia be included by others, it becomes increasingly unlikely that they will be able to manage this for themselves and a state of depression and vegetation may occur.

Inclusion is about being in or being brought into the social world, either physically or verbally. It relates to facilitating engagement where there would otherwise be none, and making a person feel they are part of the group, and are welcomed and accepted. Recognising people's worth, including them in discussions and activities emphasising a sense of belonging, and having fun together all support the need for people to feel included. Stigmatising, ignoring, banishment and mockery undermine the need for inclusion being met.

> Your name, the label that belongs to you, often is not there. Your face is familiar somehow but meeting you happens too quickly for me to search through my disjointed memory and find a label for you or a context of why I know you. I need time and clues, not questions. Try to chat about shared experiences so that I can find out why I know you, then maybe your label will appear. I realised something quite important about the way I recognise people. I would see a face and know it well and there would be a spark of recognition, and of joy in knowing. I would then smile and hug these dear people for I knew they loved me for who I am. (Bryden 2005, p.109)

What it might feel like to have personhood undermined or supported

Below are two pieces of prose taken from *Dementia Reconsidered* by Tom Kitwood. The first is imagining what the internal world might feel like for a person with dementia living in a care setting where personhood was undermined.

> You are in a swirling fog, and in half-darkness. You are wandering around in a place that seems vaguely familiar; and yet you do not know where you are; you cannot make out whether it is summer or winter, day or night. At times the fog clears a little, and you can see a few objects really clearly; but as soon as you start to get your bearings, you are overpowered by a kind of dullness and stupidity; your knowledge slips away, and again you are utterly confused.
>
> While you are stumbling in the fog, you have an impression of people rushing past you, chattering like baboons. They seem to be so energetic and purposeful, but their business is incomprehensible. Occasionally you pick up fragments of conversation, and have the impres-

sion that they are talking about you. Sometimes you catch sight of a familiar place; but as you move towards the face it vanishes, or turns into a demon. You feel desperately lost, alone, bewildered and frightened. In this dreadful state you find that you cannot control your bladder, or your bowels; you are completely losing your grip; you feel dirty, guilty, ashamed; it's so unlike how you used to be, that you don't even know yourself.

And then there are the interrogations. Official people ask you to perform strange tasks which you cannot fully understand; such as counting backwards from one hundred, or obeying the instruction 'if you are over 50 put your hands above your head'. You are never told the purpose or the results of these interrogations. You'd be willing to help, eager to co-operate, if only you knew what it was all about, and if someone took you seriously enough to guide you.

This is present reality: everything is falling apart, nothing gets completed, nothing makes sense. Behind the fog and the darkness there is a vague memory of good times, when you knew where and who you were, when you felt close to others, and when you were able to perform daily tasks with skill and grace; once the sun shone brightly and the landscape of life had richness and pattern. But now all that has been vandalised, ruined, and you are left in chaos, carrying the terrible sense of loss that can never be made good. Once you were a person who counted; now you are nothing, and good for nothing. A sense of oppression hangs over you, intensifying at times into naked terror; its meaning is that you might be abandoned for ever, left to rot and disintegrate into un-being.

Taken from Kitwood, T. (1997) *Dementia Reconsidered.* Buckingham: Open University Press, p. 77. This material is re-produced with the kind permission of The Open University Press/McGraw-Hill Publishing Company.

The second is what life could be like if care was truly person-centred.

You are in a garden, at the start of a summer's day. The air is warm and gentle, carrying the sweet scent of flowers, and a slight mist is floating around. You can't make out the shape of everything, but you are aware of some beautiful colours, blue, orange, pink and purple; the grass is green as emerald. You don't know where you are, but this doesn't matter. You somehow feel 'at home', and there is a sense of harmony and peace.

As you walk around, you become aware of other people. Several of them seem to know you; it is a joy to be greeted so warmly, and by name. There are one or two of them whom you feel sure you know well. And then there is that one special person. She seems so warm, so kind, so understanding. She must be your mother; how good it is to be back with her again. The flame of life now burns brightly and cheerfully within you. It hasn't always been like this. Somewhere, deep inside, there are dim memories of times of crushing loneliness and ice-cold fear. When that was, you do not know; perhaps it was in another life. Now there is company whenever you want it, and quietness when that is what you prefer. This is the place where you belong, with these wonderful people; they are like a kind of family.

The work that you do here is the best that you have ever had. The hours are flexible, and the job is pleasant; being with people is what you have always enjoyed. You can do the work at exactly your own pace, without any rush or pressure, and you can rest whenever you need. For instance there is a kind man who often comes to see you – by a strange coincidence his name is the same as that of your husband. He seems to need you, and to enjoy being with you. You, for your part, are glad to give time to being with him, his presence, strangely, gives you comfort.

As you pass a mirror you catch a glimpse of a person who looks quite old. Is it your grandmother or that person who used to live next door? Anyway, it is good to see her too. Then you begin to feel tired: you find a chair and you sit down, alone. Soon you become aware of a chill around your heart, a sinking feeling in your stomach – the deadly fear is coming over you again. You are about to cry out, but then you see that kind mother-person, already there, sitting beside you. Her hand is held out towards you, waiting for you to grasp it. As you talk together, the fear evaporates like the morning mist, and you are again in the garden, relaxing in the golden warmth of the sun. You know it isn't heaven itself, but sometimes it feels as if it might be half way there.

Taken from Kitwood, T. (1997) *Dementia Reconsidered*. Buckingham: Open University Press, pp. 84–5. This material is reproduced with the kind permission of The Open University Press/McGraw-Hill Publishing Company.

Putting supportive social environments into practice

What follows is a series of questions to help your organisation reflect on where you are in terms of the Supportive Social Environment element of person-centred care.

As with the Personal Perspectives element, the indicators in the Supportive Social Environment element of VIPS primarily need to be led by those who are responsible for the day-to-day management of direct care staff and the direct service environment. These indicators are about the way in which direct care staff respond to those they care for, and the skills and values they have in their communication with service users.

As I said in the last chapter, having responsibility for the direct day-to-day management of a service, or leading shifts within a service, is a tough job, and prioritising the interpersonal care is a real challenge when there are so many other competing calls on your time.

One of the ways that can put this higher up the agenda for a care provider is using a tool such as Dementia Care Mapping (DCM) to highlight strengths and needs in this important element of person-centred care.

Kitwood wrote, 'Both the according of personhood and the failure to do so, have consequences that are empirically testable' (Kitwood 1997a, p.8).

The empirical testing he was referring to here was the development of DCM. Although some of his writing and ideas may have been difficult to grasp by those providing direct care, the creation of DCM provides a means of concrete feedback on the quality of the social environment. Many of the indicators in this section cannot be examined without a direct observation of care.

What follows is a series of questions to help your organisation benchmark where you are in terms of the Supportive Social Environments element of person-centred care. These questions help to identify whether organisations have the skills and resources to provide supportive care.

---

1. Inclusion

Are people with dementia helped by staff to be included in conversations and helped to relate to others? Is there an absence of people being 'talked across'?

One of the most frequently observed of all the Personal Detractions in DCM is ignoring. A typical example of this would be two care workers having a conversation, possibly about the care needs of an individual who is sat between them, with no reference or attempt to include the person with dementia at all. At a basic level of MSP, unless efforts are made for this not to happen, staff treat the people they care for as if they simply are not there.

In some care services, people with dementia are seen as part of the furniture – to be vacuumed around, tidied up and polished – but not to be communicated with. This is true in many service settings where people are cared for, let alone those service settings for people with dementia. Think about the way that people waiting to be seen in Accident and Emergency departments are known as 'chairs', or people waiting to be discharged from hospital are 'bed-blockers'.

In order for people to get their needs for attachment and inclusion met, staff will often need to play an active role in ensuring that people are encouraged to take part in the social network of life. Staff have an active role in helping someone feel included on many levels. This might be by physically helping them move to somewhere where they can see others and be at the centre of the action, or it might be in knowing key stories from their life and prompting their use in conversation.

This aspect of MSP is difficult to eradicate, so services that do manage it well are to be applauded. In a DCM evaluation, a service that is doing well on this indicator would show low levels of stigmatisation, withholding, labelling, disempowerment, imposition, disruption, objectification and ignoring. If inclusion was part of routine care, then within a DCM evaluation you would expect to see evidence of acknowledgement, genuineness, validation, recognition, including, belonging and fun. General emotional well-being and engagement would be expected to be better in environments where people feel a sense of belonging rather than being marginalised.

It can also be evidenced by interviews with staff, service users, and their family and friends.

---

2. Respect

Are all service users treated with respect with an absence of people being demeaned by 'tellings off' or labelling?

Treating a person with respect and courtesy indicates a powerful message that we see the person as a valued member of society and that we hold them in esteem. We enter into a relationship with someone we respect based on an attitude of acceptance and positive regard. We recognise them, remember them and take delight in their skills and achievements.

When there is not a culture of respect for the person with dementia, then there is a tendency for them to be infantilised by care workers and treated in a patronising way, being told off or disparaged as if they were a naughty child. In an atmosphere of no respect, their shortcomings will be labelled and they may even be referred to as them – such as a smearer or a shouter.

If people feel respected, they are more likely to show respect for themselves and for those around them. A culture of respect would be evidenced in a DCM evaluation by high levels of signs of respect, acceptance and celebration. High levels of in-fantilisation, labelling and disparagement would indicate that this is not a respectful environment. In a care environment that is respectful and accepting, one would expect a higher overall inci-dence of well-being than in an environment where people feel put-down or incompetent.

---

3. Warmth

Is there an atmosphere of warmth and acceptance to service users? Do people look comfortable or intimidated and neglected?

Warmth or an unconditional positive regard is at the heart of a supportive social psychology that helps people particularly to feel comfortable, confident and at ease. If I do not feel welcome and wanted by those around me, then my personhood shrivels. Is the service marked by smiles, genuine concern and helpful-ness? Do staff demonstrate affection, care and concern for service users? Do they create a relaxed atmosphere by the pace of communication with service users?

On the other hand, is there evidence of staff not providing attention when it is asked for? Are information and choices presented at a rate that is too fast for people to follow? Confrontation is another common response in staff teams who do not understand the nature of dementia, or who are working in a culture of blame.

If people feel at ease in a service setting, this will be evidenced by relaxed body posture and the confidence to communicate with others.

This would be evidenced in a DCM evaluation by high levels of warmth, holding and a relaxed pace. High levels of intimidation, withholding and outpacing would indicate that this is not a warm environment. In a care environment that is warm and accepting, one would expect a higher overall incidence of well-being than in an environment where people feel tense and intimidated.

---

4. Validation

Are people's fears taken seriously? Are people left alone for long periods in emotional distress?

Validation is the recognition and the supporting of the reality of another person, and having particular sensitivity to the feelings and emotional state of that person. There is a genuine concern to understand and acknowledge the feelings of service users. The emotional state is accepted and people are not blamed or made to feel stupid for the way they feel.

If people feel that their emotional needs are respected and understood, they are more likely to be in a state of better emotional well-being over time. If distress is met promptly and empathically, then it is likely to dissipate more quickly than if people spend long periods of time in unattended emotional distress.

This would be evidenced in a DCM evaluation by high levels of signs of validation, genuineness and acknowledgement. High levels of invalidation, treachery and accusation would indicate that this is a non-validating environment. In a care environment that is validating of people's emotions, one would expect a higher overall incidence of well-being and less challenging behaviour than in an environment where people feel at sea with their distress.

---

5. Enabling

Do staff help people with dementia to be active in their own care and activity? Is there an absence of people being treated like objects with no feelings?

Enabling means identifying and encouraging someone's level of engagement within a frame of reference. It is very easy in busy care environments to take over a person with dementia completely: to feed them, to dress them, to wash them without enabling them to do the parts of these routines that they can for themselves. Not allowing people to use the abilities that they have is disempowering in the extreme.

The amount of support that individuals need with their own care will vary over time. The right amount of support will enable someone to feel empowered. Too little support will result in people feeling anxious and overwhelmed. Too much support can make people feel angry and stupid. The staff skills of facilitation – assessing the level of support required and providing the right amount – and the skill of collaboration – treating someone as a full and equal partner in what is happening, consulting and working with them – are critical if enabling is to occur.

At the extreme are care environments where people are disabled when they make an attempt to do anything. In these environments, a person's wish to do something is over-ridden. This has been particularly evident in the response to some care providers to so-called 'wandering'. Walking about has been seen as a problem behaviour to be stopped. Where this is the mind set, restraint, confrontation and disempowerment occur on a regular basis. Restraint may include physically restraining people in chairs or beds, which is an accepted practice in many parts of the world. It may also include blocking people in by use of chairs or other obstacles. It may include the use of cot-sides to prevent people getting out of bed. There are occasions where the risk of falling is such a concern that a plan of care has to be in place to protect the well-being of a particular service user. The use of restraint, however, as a first line of response is not conducive to a positive social environment for someone who has the urge to walk and who can see no reason why they should not do so.

It may also include chemical restraint where there is a high reliance on neuroleptic medication to sedate people.

This can be evidenced by care plan audit, medication audit and observation of practice.

If people feel enabled to do things rather than prevented from following their desires, they are more likely to be in a state of better emotional well-being over time. Their general levels of activity and engagement are likely to be higher. This would be evidenced in a DCM evaluation by high levels of well-being and activity, and by Personal Enhancers such as empowerment, facilitation, enabling and collaboration. High levels of disempowerment, imposition, disruption and objectification would indicate a disempowering social environment.

6. Part of the community

Is there evidence of service users using local community facilities and people from the local community visiting regularly?

Although many of the large institutions where people with dementia lived for many years have closed down in the UK to be replaced with community facilities, the lived experience of institutionalisation is alive and well in the care of people with dementia. Although nursing homes and residential homes may be smaller than the old Victorian asylums, the idea of the closed institution where people never leave the building or grounds remains. Many people never get to put on a hat and a coat and outdoor shoes, to go on a bus or to visit the pub, shop or place of worship. These are the activities that people take as part of ordinary life. They help us to maintain our identity and our interest in life in all its variety. People with dementia need this variety as much as anyone else. Likewise, services that support people in their own homes are often seen as a 'sitting-service' rather than a service that enables people to remain part of their community.

Also, there are many nursing homes and residential homes where no one from the local community has ever stepped inside. Some places are still seen as if they have the large brick wall built around them that used to surround the old asylums. Places that encourage visitors also encourage life. There are many innovative schemes of therapists, artists and hobbyists visiting with residents. There is much that can be done by local friends and volunteers. Having a bar that is open to people from outside, or a nursery or play scheme sharing some of the communal facilities, can help people maintain a sense of involvement in ordinary life and break down some of the stigma surrounding dementia.

These sorts of activities and events can be evidenced by an audit of activities and visitors as well as by interviews and questionnaires with staff and visitors.

Summary

Element Four of person-centred care is about providing care that supports people in relationships with others, and helps them to remain part of the human club and involved in life. The lived experience of care is one where people feel secure, welcomed, validated and enabled through good communication and inclusive practice. Services are part of the community in its truest sense rather than mini-institutions.

6

Care in Context

The term 'person-centred care' was first used by Kitwood to differentiate ways of working with people with dementia that were not framed within a biological or technical model. Understanding and expertise in the provision of person-centred care have developed enormously since the term was first used.

This book is an attempt to articulate the different elements of person-centred care and to describe what these look like in practice. The list of elements and indicators should be seen as work in progress rather than a definition set in stone. The elements and indicators come from my experience of working in care practice in the UK and of visiting services around the world that are trying to provide humanising care, as well as my knowledge of the evidence base for what works in dementia care. I also have the privilege of working in a job where I have time to reflect on these issues in depth. The initial VIPS indicators were developed a couple of years ago. Approximately 50 service providers in the UK and the USA piloted the original tool and provided feedback. This has helped to refine the final indicators that have been set out in the chapters here.

It is interesting to consider whether this definition might work as a model to facilitate some predictions of what might happen if only certain elements of person-centred care are in place while others are neglected. The following observations are again based on experience of working with many care facilities for people with dementia. They are summarised diagrammatically in Figure 6.1.

Under-emphasis of this element	Element	Emphasis placed only on this element but not others
Discrimination within care organisations and policy agenda against people with dementia and those who care for them.	V	Care evangelism. Platitudes that people agree with but don't know how to put into practice.
Chaotic and inappropriate assessments and care plans for people with complex needs and life histories.	I	Lots of paperwork. Care plans are all different from each other but meet individual needs only within a narrow range.
Care will not meet the priorities of the individual. High levels of challenging behaviour and learned helplessness.	P	Lots of information collected but never used appropriately.
Poor communication and lack of dementia-aware interpersonal skills by staff. Organisational emphasis on safety and aesthetics.	S	Slavish following of techniques. Frequent changes in direction as latest techniques are tried and discarded.

Figure 6.1: Towards a model of person-centred care for people with dementia

The first part of the model (V) is valuing anti-discriminatory practice for people with dementia and those who work with them. The push for anti-dementia-ism, however, has largely come from people with dementia themselves, their families and those who work in the field. It is not explicit in the value statements of many care organisations or in government policy. The danger in not making it explicit is that the pressures of dementia-ism are so powerful in society that they will erode attempts at person-centred care that are not firmly built on a strategy of positively valuing individuals with dementia within the context of care. Valuing people with dementia is something that care providers have to be actively signed up to if they are to implement person-centred care.

On the other hand, if person-centred care is seen *only* as a value base, then it can quickly become seen as a group of empty words or evangelism without a practical application and a body of knowledge. There are some people who can extrapolate practice very easily from a value base, but many others need the implications to be spelt out in rather more concrete terms.

The second element (I) is the focus on the individual. If person-centred care is just taken to mean individualised care without the other elements of the definition, then care can quickly deteriorate into serving the needs within a very narrow frame that makes very little difference to the lived experience of dementia. Taking an individualised approach to care will usually entail trying to see the world from the perspective of the person with dementia. However, it is possible to do individualised assessments and care without considering the viewpoint of the person with dementia at all. In these cases, the assessment would generally focus on constructs entirely determined by the professional perspective. All service users may have individual care plans that are different from each other but may not prioritise the things that are important for each individual in any way.

On the other hand, if the practicalities of complex individual needs are not assessed and catered for, then the provision of person-centred care becomes too chaotic to be deliverable.

The third element (P) is about taking the perspective of the person with dementia as the starting point. If this is all that person-centred care is taken to mean, then a lot of information is generated that never makes a difference to people's lives. Filing cabinets in care facilities around the world are full of information about people's lives but still care staff will not know even the rudimentary facts. Individuals' perspectives need to be used if they are to be part of person-centred care.

On the other hand, without the personal perspective, care becomes little more than guesswork. The level of challenging behaviour is likely to be high as people with dementia struggle to make themselves heard. Alternatively, people may have burnt out in their attempts, and a situation of learnt helplessness develops.

The fourth element (S) is the positive social environment. These are the interpersonal skills and the individual and organisational wherewithal to make an impact on the lives of people with dementia. If this is all that person-centred care consists of, however, then there is a danger that care becomes mechanistic without reference to individual needs and perspectives. Without a strong value base, the reason for using these tools in the first place becomes obscured and a slavish following of technique can occur.

On the other hand, if care workers, family members and organisations do not have the skills and techniques to provide a positive social environment for people with dementia, then confusion and distress will reign. The organisation is likely to place an emphasis on care practice that promotes the safety of property and residents, and on the aesthetics of the physical care environment.

Summary

Dementia is a devastating problem and by looking at it in this way I am not trying to make little of the pain and the distress it causes. However, it may be that by taking a more person-centred approach to our care we can avoid some of the suffering that is caused by an absence of care that maintains personhood.

This VIPS framework does not apply just to services for people living with dementia. It applies to all who find themselves in a state of dependence and vulnerability. In other words, it applies to every single one of us. In assessing the person-centredness of an organisation, however, if they get services sorted for people with dementia and their families, there is an excellent chance that it will be good for everyone else too.

Part 2
The VIPS Framework

The VIPS Framework: Person-Centred Care for People with Dementia

Using the VIPS Framework

The VIPS definition of person-centred care encompasses four major elements:

V A value base that asserts the absolute value of all human lives regardless of age or cognitive ability.

I An individualised approach, recognising uniqueness.

P Understanding the world from the perspective of the service user.

S Providing a social environment that supports psychological needs.

These elements have been decribed in great detail in Part 1 of this book. In Part 2 the VIPS Framework Tool is presented.

This tool is designed to help care providers of services for people with dementia to assess the relative strengths and weaknesses with regard to providing person-centred care. It details six key indicators under each element that demonstrate person-centred care. For each indicator, you are asked to reflect on how your organisation is performing. You can then use this to derive an action plan for service quality improvements. In order for you to develop practice, it is helpful to complete the document as a group, preferably by people who have different roles within your organisation. It is unlikely that one person will be able to answer it all.

I use the term 'care providers' in the broadest sense. It covers all those providing a service for people with dementia in their own homes, in day care, in residential care or in health and hospital care. For each indicator, care providers are asked to reflect on how well they think they are doing on a scale of:

Excellent: This is where the care provider has no doubt they are reaching the highest standards within the indicator, they have maintained this over a period of time and it is consistent across their whole service.

Good: This is where the care provider is sure they have achieved a high standard against the indicator but they have some concerns about the consistency or sustainability of the standard in some areas of their service.

OK: This is an adequate performance that means they can provide evidence of the indicator being met most of the time, or they have elements of good practice that could be introduced more widely across the organisation.

Need to work on this: This is where the care provider does not know how they are doing on a particular indicator, where they are concerned that they have not addressed it, or where they need to identify the blocks to its being met on a consistent basis.

The VIPS framework can be used on at least three different levels:

1. **Raising awareness of person-centred care across the organisation**. Using it in this way, a group leader uses the questions to facilitate a discussion about each question. The composition of the group will depend on the size of the care organisation and the main aim in bringing people together. This could be a naturally occurring team such as a ward team, a home care team or the executive board of a care provider. It is probably most useful, however, to have a group of around 10–12 people who work at different levels within the organisation or who have responsibility for different areas. The discussion will generate many things in its own right. There will be areas to celebrate where the organisation can recognise things that it already does well and may want to publicise these further. There will be other areas where there is a mismatch of experience between different group members.

Sometimes this occurs in the difference between what is meant to happen according to policies and procedures and what actually happens in reality. There may be variation across the organisation suggesting that effective practice needs to be shared. There will be other areas where the group identifies gaps in provision and may generate an initial discussion of how this could be addressed. This sort of group facilitation needs skilful handling to ensure participants are comfortable in sharing information and in challenging each other's assumptions.

2. **Evidence collection and benchmarking**. This would be a more formal means of using the framework to actually check out how practice actually measures up in reality. Most organisations think they are doing better than they actually are! Ways of evidencing could include reviewing paper-work and records, interviewing staff and service users, focus groups on particular topics, questionnaires, observation of practice, and monitoring key indicators and critical incidents. This sort of evidence collection and analysis requires skills in evaluation and audit.

3. **Action planning for improvements in key elements**. It may be that an organisation needs to focus on one or two areas to really make an impact on practice. This might be in terms of particular working groups or learning sets coming together on specific elements or indicators. The indicators can be used to identify the key areas of concern. Using the indicators in this way requires skills in project management and practice development.

Person centred-care requires sign-up to working in this way across the whole care provider organisation if it is to be sustained over any length of time. Particular elements require leadership at different levels.

The first element – Valuing People – requires leadership from those responsible for leading the organisation at a senior level.

The second element – Individualised Care – requires leadership particularly from those responsible for setting care standards and procedures within the care organisation.

The final two elements – Personal Perspectives, and Supportive Social Environment – require leadership from those responsible for the day-to-day management and provision of care.

The VIPS Framework Reflection Points and Evidence

Name of care provider .... Date..

Type of organisation ....

Valuing: Valuing people with cognitive disabilities and those who care for them

Promoting citizenship rights and entitlements regardless of age or cognitive impairment, and rooting out discriminatory practice.

Indicator	How are we doing?
V1 VISION	
Is there a vision and mission statement about providing care that is person-centered?	
Reflection points: An organisation's mission statement spells out its reason for being and its purpose. Valuing people has to begin at the top. Valuing the equality of all regardless of age and cognitive disability is a challenge that is difficult to achieve. It is impossible to achieve fully unless those at board or trustee level do not take it as underpinning all their decisions. Agreeing this in its vision or mission statement means that the organisation is making public its policy of promoting the rights of people with dementia.	
Written material about the service provided should be available, is accessible to all service users and provided in a timely manner. It should include a vision statement about people being supported by the service regardless of their age or level of cognitive ability and how this is achieved. This information should also be available in spoken and other formats where appropriate.	Excellent Good OK Needs more work
This purpose should be clear to all members of staff at all levels from front-line to board level. It should also be clear to service users and their families and to all who come into contact with the service.	
This can be evidenced by:	
• an audit of materials available to service users about the service • staff surveys • service users' surveys and interviews • family and supporters' surveys and interviews admissions or new service user pathways.	

Indicator	How are we doing?
V2 HUMAN RESOURCE MANAGEMENT Are systems in place to ensure staff feel valued by their employers? **Reflection points**: If staff are to see communication, integrity and nurturing as important in their work with people with dementia, then this should be their experience of how the organisation relates to them as workers. Is there a recognition of the importance of building teams that work well together and are united in their purpose? Teams that see value in working together are more likely to promote a sense of shared community with all the service users in their facility, with less risk of scapegoating those people who do not fit in easily. Is there a whistle-blowing policy? How is sickness managed? What sort of induction, appraisal and reward systems exist? What are the terms and conditions of employment? How is workplace stress managed? Providing person-centred dementia care is emotionally labour intensive. How is it identified when a team is in need of extra support? What form does extra support take? How is it accessed? How is it reviewed? Is there a system of debriefing and reflection following particularly stressful events? **This can be evidenced by**: • staff surveys and interviews • audit of procedures • external accreditation – such as Investors in People.	Excellent Good OK Needs more work

Indicator	How are we doing?
V3 MANAGEMENT ETHOS Are management practices empowering to staff delivering direct care? **Reflection points**: Staff who feel their ideas for good practice are met with enthusiasm are more likely to react positively to ideas and challenges from service users. If a 'can do' culture exists for staff, they are more likely to promote this with service users and families. Markers of this might include clear avenues for communication that are used frequently between different levels of the organisation. Is there a consultation process that is trusted throughout the organisation? Staff who feel that they have been consulted over practice are more likely to institute consultation practices with families and service users. Is there an 'open door' management practice? Staff who feel that they can approach their managers if they have a problem that they cannot resolve, or an idea that will improve practice, are more likely to encourage and listen to ideas from families and service users. Is there delegation of resource management to the optimum level to provide person-centred care? Without the ability to communicate effectively with each other, the basis for providing an adequate social environment is flawed. In the absence of good communication, paranoia, confusion and anxiety flourish. This is true both for staff teams and for people in care. How are things communicated between members of staff? Is adequate time provided for handovers and communal problem-solving? Who talks to whom? What is the communication like within a shift? What is the communication like between front-line and senior staff? What is communication like between shifts, between night and day staff, between staff working in different sections of the same building? Is the communication two-way? Do people feel listened to and have the chance to have their say? **This can be evidenced by**: • staff surveys and interviews • audit of procedures, staff meetings • complaints analysis.	Excellent Good OK Needs more work

Indicator	How are we doing?
V4 TRAINING AND STAFF DEVELOPMENT Are there practices in place to support development of a workforce skilled in person-centred care? **Reflection points**: Maintaining person-centred care over time for people with dementia is not an easy or trivial process. Dementia services do not have a tradition of skilled care and the practices that are required to maintain it. There should be a recognition in your organisation that caring for people with dementia is skilled work that is emotionally and physically labour intensive. What is the training and education strategy? What is available at induction regarding working with people with dementia? How are training needs identified? What specialist courses are available? How is learning supported in the workplace? What is the level of expertise of more senior people? Have they got accredited qualifications in gerontology or dementia studies? Are there opportunities for reflective practice, supervision and mentoring? When individual practitioners or staff teams are feeling out of their depth in working with a particular service user or family, how is more expert help accessed? **This can be evidenced by**: • staff surveys and interviews • training records • skills analysis • critical incident analysis.	Excellent Good OK Needs more work

Indicator	How are we doing?
V5 SERVICE ENVIRONMENTS Are there supportive and inclusive physical and social environments for people with cognitive disability? **Reflection points**: Anti-discriminatory practice means that people with dementia have the same rights as everyone else; it does not mean that people with dementia do not need extra help in everyday life. For example, we would expect that those in wheelchairs have a right to enter buildings, and would provide elevators or ramps to help them to achieve this. Likewise, we would expect that a person with dementia has the right to find their way around the building with clear signage and way-finding markers. At a corporate level, that means that there should be evidence that this is taken into consideration in design briefs for buildings and fixtures and fittings. In the general physical design, are features such as clear colours, way-finding memory markers, unambiguous surfaces to walk on, easy access to a safe outdoor environment, natural light, low numbers of blind corners, no obvious locked doors and unobtrusive use of technology maximised to provide a non-confusing low anxiety-provoking environment? It should also ensure that all front-line staff are comfortable communicating with people with dementia. Is it policy that all staff having direct service-user contact are aware of how to help someone with dementia feel at ease? Is this evidenced in staff induction and training? **This can be evidenced by**: • service users' and carers' interviews and surveys • physical environment audits • training records • skills analysis • observation of practice.	Excellent Good OK Needs more work

Indicator	How are we doing?
V6 QUALITY ASSURANCE Are Continuous Quality Improvement mechanisms in place that are driven by knowing and acting upon needs and concerns of service users? **Reflection points**: Knowing how service users feel about the service they receive on an ongoing basis is central to person-centred care. How does your organisation know and act upon the views of service users? Does it undertake regular satisfaction surveys, interviews, focus groups, reference groups or observation of practice such as Dementia Care Mapping? Are the views of all service users regardless of level of cognitive impairment taken into account in this process, or just the most vocal? Involving service users and knowing their views is central to person-centred care – or any customer care activity. In the dementia care field this can take place through residents' groups, carers' groups, user forums and other ad hoc reference groups. How are these organised? How often do they occur? Whose responsibility are they? What happens to the views or decisions made at these meetings? Are they seen as central to the decision-making process or are they just an add-on? **This can be evidenced by**: • service users' and carers' interviews and surveys • audit of quality procedures and meetings • results of quality surveys and review • external quality assurance accreditation • training records • skills analysis • observation of practice.	Excellent Good OK Needs more work

POINTS FOR ACTION	OVERALL PERFORMANCE ON VALUING

Individualised Care: Treating people as individuals

Appreciating that all people have a unique history and personality, physical and mental health, and social and economic resources, and that these will affect their response to cognitive disabilities.

Indicator	How are we doing?
I 1 CARE PLANNING Do you identify strengths and vulnerabilities across a wide range of needs, and have individualised care plans that reflect a wide range of strengths and needs? **Reflection points**: Individualised assessment and analysis sets a basis from which interventions can be designed for both enhancing well-being by appropriately matching activity and occupation to persons with dementia, or reducing disturbed mood or behaviour. Knowing about life history, personality, lifestyle, health, cognitive support needs and capacity are all important in producing the optimal plan of care. Other interacting factors are likely to require taking into consideration such as level of dependency and a range of socio-economic, gender, ethnic or cultural differences. **This can be evidenced by**: • service users' and carers' interviews and surveys • observation of practice • assessment and care plan audit • individual care pathways and case tracking.	Excellent Good OK Needs more work

Indicator	How are we doing?
I 2 REGULAR REVIEWS Are individual care plans reviewed on a regular basis? **Reflection points**: The needs of people with dementia change over time. This is true for all of us, but particularly when working with progressive conditions we can be sure that change will occur. The pace of change will vary on an individual basis. For some the pace will be slow and insidious, so much so that it is easy to overlook subtle problems that may be causing a sense of failure in the person with dementia. For this reason, it is important that there is a fail-safe procedure so that everyone's care plan gets looked at, at least every six months to ensure that it is still meeting needs. On the other hand, there will be people whose needs change very quickly either because of the nature of their dementia or because of some other unstable physical health condition. Structures should be in place that care plans can be reviewed quickly when necessary. Building good relationships with local mental health teams or specialist services can help ensure that health and well-being are maintained at the optimal level. They can be useful where there are issues of significant deterioration, worsening confusion or depression. **This can be evidenced by**: • service users' and carers' interviews and surveys • assessment and care plan audit • care pathways and case tracking.	Excellent Good OK Needs more work

Indicator	How are we doing?
I 3 PERSONAL POSSESSIONS Do service users have their own personal clothing and possessions for everyday use? **Reflection points**: As dementia progresses, people will obtain much greater comfort from wearing clothes that look familiar and using objects that are well known, rather than getting to grips with new purchases. The reasons for this are two-fold. First, familiar items are a touchstone in a world that feels increasingly alien to people living with dementia. It links the present with the past, the unfamiliar with the known. Second, as dementia progresses, people often lose the ability to learn how to use new objects quickly, whereas with old objects the patterns are well learnt. Most of us have the experience of turning on a lamp with which we are familiar without even consciously thinking about where the switch is. With a new lamp, we have to stop and think. It is the latter action that becomes difficult to manage in dementia. Surround the person with things that are familiar and they will be more at ease. When new things need to be purchased, try to buy the same make or model, or buy clothes in the same material as ones that were cherished. **This can be evidenced by**: • service users' and carers' interviews and surveys • observation of practice • assessment and care plan audit • care pathways and case tracking.	 Excellent Good OK Needs more work

Indicator	How are we doing?
I 4 INDIVIDUAL PREFERENCES Are individual likes and dislikes, preferences and daily routines known about by direct care staff and acted upon? **Reflection points**: If familiar objects are important in dementia care, then familiar foods, drinks, music and routines are even more so. Familiarity with day-to-day experiences help to establish security, trust and comfort. As anxiety decreases, so will the likelihood that a person will try to 'go home' in an attempt to find the familiar. People with dementia are very vulnerable to feeling culturally isolated. If any of us are feeling vulnerable, then familiar touchstones of our cultural identity, our spirituality or religion, and food and drinks and music with which we are familiar are likely to have a calming effect. Vulnerability, anxiety and alienation are more likely to increase if those elements are missing. There is an increasing recognition that trying to ensure there is a familiarity in long-held routines and preferences is an important way of helping people feel at ease. Sometimes people will be able to tell us about these routines and preferences for themselves. Others will not, which is when getting this information from family and friends can be useful. Do direct care staff know food and drink preference, clothing preferences, bathing and hygiene routines, work routines, hobbies, favourite music, sports and people? **This can be evidenced by**: • service users' and carers' interviews and surveys • observation of practice • assessment and care plan audit • care pathways and case tracking.	Excellent Good OK Needs more work

Indicator	How are we doing?
I 5 LIFE HISTORY Are care staff aware of basic individual life histories and key stories of proud times, and are these used regularly? **Reflection points:** As dementia progresses, it becomes more difficult to hold on to the stories of one's life and to be able to tell others of the defining moments that shaped one's identity. One of the jobs of caring for someone with dementia is to learn these key stories and hold this narrative for them. This can be used to improve self-esteem and to maintain an identity in the face of increasing confusion. As the capacity for engagement becomes more difficult, objects that trigger good feelings become increasingly important. Past experiences of vulnerability and trauma, particularly those that happened in childhood or teenage years, can often be relived during a dementia illness which may have emotional resonance with these past experiences. For example, if someone has a history of being sexually abused, they may find help with personal care activities particularly traumatic. Understanding a person's past history and using this knowledge in direct care is crucial to providing person-centred care for people with dementia. This can be evidenced around looking at procedures for how key stories are known about and how these are communicated. Knowing whether they are used by staff in everyday situations requires observation of practice. **This can be evidenced by:** • service users' and carers' interviews and surveys • observation of practice • assessment and care plan audit • individual care pathways and case tracking.	Excellent Good OK Needs more work

Indicator	How are we doing?
I 6 ACTIVITY AND OCCUPATION	
Are there a variety of activities available to meet the needs and abilities of all service users?	
Reflection points: Boredom and lack of meaningful activity is rife in institutional care for older people generally, but particularly those with dementia who often find it difficult to initiate or sustain activities. Finding things that interest and sustain people can be a challenge. As well as knowing what is meaningful to each individual, understanding the capabilities of individuals with regard to their level or severity of dementia is likely to be important for providing suitable activities. In the early stages, cognitive therapies or goal-directed activities such as competitive games or crafts might be most productive. Behavioural interventions or creative therapies might be most therapeutic in the middle stages of dementia while sensory stimulation might be most appropriate for people with the highest levels of cognitive and functional impairment.	
How this can be achieved in long-term care settings or by people living with dementia at home requires careful consideration. Who has responsibility for ensuring that service users have access to fun and meaningful activity on a day-to-day basis? How is this provided? How is it monitored to ensure it meets the needs of individuals? In any institutional service setting, there has to be an appreciation that all staff from direct care workers through to management share in the responsibility for the provision of fun and occupation that gives meaning and structure to life and staves off boredom.	Excellent Good OK Needs more work
This can be evidenced by:	
• service users' and carers' interviews and surveys • observation of practice • assessment and care plan audit • individual care pathways and case tracking.	

POINTS FOR ACTION	OVERALL PERFORMANCE ON INDIVIDU-ALISED CARE

Personal Perspective: Looking at the world from the perspective of the person with dementia

Recognising that each person's experience has its own psychological validity, that people with cognitive disabilities act from this perspective, and that empathy with this perspective has its own therapeutic potential.

Indicator	How are we doing?
P1 COMMUNICATION WITH SERVICE USERS On a day-to-day basis, are service users asked for their preferences, consent and opinions? **Reflection points**: In order to know a person's opinion, it is important that they are asked directly about this! It is surprising how often, however, this basic courtesy and social interaction does not occur in services for people with dementia. Although people may lose the capacity to make truly informed choices about abstract decisions as time goes by, the evidence is that people can make reliable decisions about long-held preferences well into their dementia. Even if the capacity for understanding language is severely impaired, the non-verbal behaviour that accompanies being asked for permission or opinion will not go unnoticed and will do much to convey to the person with dementia that they are worth bothering about.	
In everyday practice, are people asked what they want to eat or drink, where they would like to sit and what they need to feel comfortable? Are attempts made to discuss these sorts of issues directly with the person with dementia? Are the direct care staff good communicators generally? Do they recognise the barriers to communication due to sensory disability and have strategies to overcome these? Do they recognise the barriers to communication due to cognitive disabilities and have strategies to overcome these?	Excellent Good OK Needs more work
When decisions need to be made that are either too complex or abstract for the service user with dementia to make an informed decision about, do staff talk to people who know them well, such as family, and who can often offer insight into their past preferences? Is this backed up by observations of the person in different situations to attempt or confirm a best estimation of their wishes? **This can be evidenced by**: • assessment and care plan audit – is the perspective of the service user represented within all paperwork relating to them? • direct observations of practice: for example in a DCM evaluation a high occurrence of Personal Enhancers such as negotiation, collaboration, enabling and respect in environments where communication is high on the agenda. There will also be evidence of a higher level of engagement overall particularly with staff.	

Indicator	How are we doing?
P2 EMPATHY and ACCEPTABLE RISK Do staff show the ability to put themselves in the position of the person they are caring for and to think about decisions from their point of view? **Reflection points**: There will be occasions where the person with dementia is unable to fully participate and put forward their own point of view. It is important then that staff are able to try to think things through from the viewpoint of the person with dementia. This may be particularly important around issues of risk assessment. There is often tremendous pressure to err on the side of caution with regards to situations that may include an element of risk. People with dementia are a vulnerable group within our society and it is wholly right that those responsible for their care work to ensure their safety. People with dementia are, however, in danger of being kept so safe that they have no quality of life at all. There are hidden dangers and risks that exist to emotional well-being, in the form of boredom, helplessness, depression and giving up. Often, it will be up to the person's key worker or a professional to advocate on behalf of their emotional well-being. In order to put this into practice, are staff able to tell if a person with dementia is in a state of relative well-being or ill-being? Can they identify, describe and respond appropriately to verbal and non-verbal signs of well- and ill-being? Is this done as part of a decision-making process about risk? **This can be evidenced by**: • auditing risk assessment documentation and care plans – it is useful to see whether decisions have been made purely on the basis of physical safety or whether attempts have been made to look at various options and activities from the point of view of the service user and their emotional well-being • observation of practice – the Personal Enhancers of relaxed pace, validation and facilitation present alongside low levels of withdrawn and distressed states would also indicate that staff are working at an empathic level.	Excellent Good OK Needs more work

Indicator	How are we doing?
P3 PHYSICAL ENVIRONMENT Is the physical environment – e.g. noise, temperature – managed on a day-to-day basis to help people with dementia feel at ease? **Reflection points**: People with dementia are often at the mercy of other people controlling their physical environment. Attention may have been paid to the physical design of such facilities – they may even have won architectural awards – but, unless the micro-environment is managed so that people are comfortable, then such endeavour is worthless. On a day-to-day basis, it is important that staff use their empathic skills to be actively aware of the comfort needs of people with dementia. Often people with dementia may not be able to tell staff directly that they are in discomfort, or they may not be able to work out for themselves how to alleviate discomfort. **This can be evidenced by**: • direct observations in care settings • environmental audits • interviews with service users and visitors.	Excellent Good OK Needs more work

Indicator	How are we doing?
P4 PHYSICAL HEALTH Are the physical health needs of people with dementia, including pain assessment, sight and hearing problems, given due attention? **Reflection points**: In recognition that people with dementia often can't describe symptoms of pain or sensory deficit, this has to be actively monitored by staff. People with dementia are prone to having physical health problems that can go undetected for a long time if staff around them are not vigilant about investigating causes of any sudden increase in confusion. When caring for a person with dementia, any sudden increase in the level of confusion should be treated with the suspicion that there could be a physical health problem contributing to the general confusion. Physical fitness and comfort needs to be taken seriously. Poor physical health greatly intensifies the impairments caused by dementia. Pain is often undetected in people with dementia and the manifestations of the person's discomfort may be misperceived as episodes of 'challenging behaviour'. As people with dementia may have difficulty remembering episodes of pain or difficulty finding the words to describe their symptoms, the onus has to be on the carers to be proactive in this respect. Unaddressed age-related sensory impairments, such as not having the correct spectacles or functioning hearing aids, often lie at the root of communication problems. If someone has poor visual perception and dysphasia due to their dementia, this only gets worse if they do not have all the help they can get from physical prostheses. Again, because of their dementia, an individual may not be able to say that they have lost their glasses or to complain that their hearing aid no longer functions. Professionals and care staff have to be vigilant on their behalf. **This can be evidenced by**: • an analysis of hospital admissions • care plan audit with particular reference to pain management • audit of glasses, hearing aids and dentures.	Excellent Good OK Needs more work

Indicator	How are we doing?
P5 CHALLENGING BEHAVIOUR AS COMMUNICATION Is 'challenging behaviour' analysed to discover the underlying reasons for it? **Reflection points**: Is an attempt made to understand heightened distress, aggression, inappropriate sexual behaviour, low mood, withdrawal and self-harm by reference to a bio-psychosocial model and care plans altered accordingly to take this into account? A person-centred response would be to see the challenge in them as one that challenges a care team to find the reasons underlying the behaviour and to help the person achieve a state of well-being. In understanding the perspective of the service user and using this as part of our detailed analysis, we can then have a plan that supports personhood. The reasons underlying challenging behaviours can usually be understood by reference to the Enriched Model of dementia. Is there something about this person's cognitive disability that means they are misinterpreting or becoming overwhelmed by their situation? Is there something in their past life that is being triggered by their current situation that is causing distress? Is there a mismatch between their preferences and needs and what the current environment is offering? Is there an untreated physical complaint that is causing an increase in confusion or pain? Is the level of social care meeting their personhood needs? **This can be evidenced by**: • case tracking and individual care pathways of a service user whose behaviour challenges the service • care plan audit • prescribing analysis and audit • interviews with service users, families and visitors.	Excellent Good OK Needs more work

Indicator	How are we doing?
P6 ADVOCACY In situations where the actions of an individual with dementia are at odds with the safety and well-being of others, how are the rights of the individual protected? **Reflection points**: The most difficult situations in long-term care settings are when the rights of one individual are at odds with the safety and comfort of others. An example of this might arise within a housing facility where a resident who is disorientated is constantly knocking on neighbours' doors. Another example could be within a residential home where a resident has become sexually disinhibited and is making sexual advances to others that are not welcomed. In such a situation, the initial response is that the person who is causing the problem should be removed to another facility. The problem with this response is that it may actually exacerbate the problem for the individual concerned and simply make it someone else's responsibility. In some cases, it may truly be the case that the individual's needs can be met better elsewhere because of better trained staff or higher staffing ratios. There is no simple solution to situations such as these but they occur with enough regularity that some mechanism for dealing with them needs to be in place before they occur. This sort of situation usually gives rise to a case conference or case review and the person who may not be able to argue their own corner should have someone advocating on their behalf. In some situations, this might be a social worker or a community nurse. In other situations, it might be that the organisation calls on the services of a formal advocacy service. **This can be evidenced by**: • case tracking and individual care pathways of a service user whose behaviour challenges the service • care plan audit • interviews with service users, families and visitors.	Excellent Good OK Needs more work

POINTS FOR ACTION	OVERALL PERFORMANCE ON SERVICE-USER PERSPECTIVE

Social Environment

Recognising that all human life is grounded in relationships and that people with cognitive disabilities need an enriched social environment which both compensates for their impairment and fosters opportunities for personal growth.

On a day-to-day basis, this relates to the knowledge, skills and qualities of staff who provide direct care to people with cognitive disabilities.

Indicator	How are we doing?
S1 INCLUSION Are people with dementia helped by staff to be included in conversations and helped to relate to others? Is there an absence of people being 'talked across'? **Reflection points:** One of the most frequently observed of all the Personal Detractions in DCM is ignoring. A typical example of this would be two care workers having a conversation, possibly about the care needs of an individual who is sitting between them, with no reference or attempt to include the person with dementia at all. At a basic level of MSP, unless efforts are made for this not to happen, staff treat the people they care for as if they simply are not there. In some care services, people with dementia are seen as part of the furniture – to be vacuumed around, tidied up and polished – but not to be communicated with. In order for people to get their needs for attachment and inclusion met, staff will often need to play an active role in ensuring that people are encouraged to take part in the social network of life. Staff have an active role in helping someone feel included on many levels. This might be by physically helping them move to somewhere where they can see others and be at the centre of the action, or it might be in knowing key stories from their life and prompting their use in conversation. **This can be evidenced by**: • observation of practice of a service that is doing well on this indicator would show low levels of stigmatisation, withholding, labelling, disempowerment, imposition, disruption, objectification and ignoring. If Inclusion was part of routine care, then you would expect to see evidence of acknowledgement, genuineness, validation, recognition, including, belonging and fun. General emotional well-being and engagement would be expected to be better in environments where people feel a sense of belonging rather than being marginalised • interviews with staff interviews with service users and family carers.	Excellent Good OK Needs more work

✓

Indicator	How are we doing?
S2 RESPECT Are all service users treated with respect, with an absence of people being demeaned by 'tellings off' or labelling? **Reflection points**: Treating a person with respect and courtesy indicates a powerful message that we see the person as a valued member of society and that we hold them in esteem. We enter into a relationship with someone we respect based on an attitude of acceptance and positive regard. We recognise them, remember them and take delight in their skills and achievements. When there is not a culture of respect for the person with dementia, then there is a tendency for them to be infantilised by care workers, for them to be treated in a patronising way, being told off or disparaged as if they were a naughty child. In an atmosphere of no respect, their shortcomings will be labelled and they may even be referred to as them – such as a smearer or a shouter. If people feel respected, they are more likely to show respect for themselves and for those around them. **This can be evidenced by**: • observation of practice: a culture of respect would be evidenced by high levels of signs of respect, acceptance and celebration. High levels of infantilisation, labelling and disparagement would indicate that this is not a respectful environment. In a care environment that is respectful and accepting, one would expect a higher overall incidence of well-being than in an environment where people feel put-down or incompetent • interviews with staff • interviews with service users and family carers.	Excellent Good OK Needs more work

Indicator	How are we doing?
S3 WARMTH Is there an atmosphere of warmth and acceptance to service users? Do people look comfortable or intimidated and neglected? **Reflection points**: Warmth or an unconditional positive regard is at the heart of a supportive social psychology that helps people feel comfortable, confident and at ease. If people do not feel welcome and wanted by those around them, then personhood shrivels. Is the service marked by smiles, genuine concern and helpfulness? Do staff demonstrate affection, care and concern for service users? Do they create a relaxed atmosphere by the pace of communication with service users? On the other hand, is there evidence of staff not providing attention when it is asked for? Are information and choices presented at a rate that is too fast for a person to follow? Confrontation is another common response in staff teams who do not understand the nature of dementia or who are working in a culture of blame. If people feel at ease in a service setting, this will be evidenced by relaxed body posture and the confidence to communicate with others. **This can be evidenced by**: • observation of practice: high levels of Personal Enhancers of warmth, holding and a relaxed pace would indicate this is a positively accepting environment whereas high levels of intimidation, withholding and outpacing would indicate the contrary. In a care environment that is warm and accepting, one would expect a higher overall incidence of well-being than in an environment where people feel tense and intimidated • interviews with staff • interviews with service users and family carers.	Excellent Good OK Needs more work

Indicator	How are we doing?
S4 VALIDATION Are people's fears taken seriously? Are people left alone for long periods in emotional distress? **Reflection points**: Validation is the recognition and the supporting of the reality of another person having particular sensitivity to feeling and the emotional state of that person. There is a genuine concern to understand and acknowledge the feelings of service users. The emotional state is accepted and people are not blamed or made to feel stupid for the way they feel. If people feel that their emotional needs are respected and understood, they are more likely to enjoy better emotional well-being over time. If distress is met promptly and empathically, then it is likely to dissipate more quickly than if people spend long periods of time in unattended emotional distress. **This can be evidenced by**: • observation of practice: this would be evidenced by high levels of signs of validation, genuineness and acknowledgement. High levels of invalidation, treachery and accusation would indicate that this is non-validating environment. In a care environment that is validating of people's emotions, one would expect a higher overall incidence of well-being and less challenging behaviour than in an environment where people feel at sea with their distress • interviews with staff • interviews with service users and family carers.	Excellent Good OK Needs more work

Indicator	How are we doing?
S5 ENABLING Do staff help people with cognitive disabilities to be active in their own care and activity? Is there an absence of people being treated like objects with no feelings? **Reflection points**: Enabling means identifying and encouraging someone's level of engagement within a frame of reference. It is very easy in busy care environments to take over a person with dementia completely: to feed them, to dress them, to wash them without enabling them to do what parts of these routines they can for themselves. Not allowing people to use the abilities that they do have is disempowering in the extreme. The amount of support that individuals need with their own care will vary over time. The right amount of support will enable someone to feel empowered. Too little support will result in people feeling anxious and overwhelmed. Too much support can make people feel angry and stupid. The staff skills of facilitation – assessing the level of support required and providing the right amount – and the skill of collaboration – treating someone as a full and equal partner in what is happening, consulting and working with them – are critical if enabling is to occur. **This can be evidenced by**: • observation of practice: high level of positive mood/low levels of distress that is unattended and a high level of engagement overall with evidence of empowerment would suggest an enabling environment. Low level of positive mood/high levels of distress and withdrawal, low level of engagement and evidence of disempowerment, imposition, disruption and objectification would suggest a non-enabling environment • interviews with staff • interviews with service users and family carers • care plan audit with particular reference to use of medication and restraint.	Excellent Good OK Needs more work

Indicator	How are we doing?
S6 PART OF THE COMMUNITY Is there evidence of service users using local community facilities and people from the local community visiting regularly? **Reflection points**: Although nursing homes and residential homes may be smaller than the old Victorian asylums, the idea of the closed institution where people never leave the building or grounds remains. Many people never get to put on a hat and a coat and outdoor shoes, to go on a bus or to visit the pub, shop or place of worship. These are the activities that people take as part of ordinary life. They help us to maintain our identity and our interest in life in all its variety. People with dementia need this variety as much as anyone else. Likewise, services that support people in their own homes are often seen as a 'sitting-service' rather than a service that enables people to remain part of their community. Also, there are many nursing homes and residential homes where no one from the local community has ever stepped inside. Some places are still seen as if they have the large brick wall built around them that used to surround the old asylums. Places that encourage visitors also encourage life. There are many innovative schemes of therapists, artists and hobbyists visiting with residents. There is much that can be done by local friends and volunteers. Having a bar that is open to people from outside, or a nursery or play scheme sharing some of the communal facilities, can help people maintain a sense of involvement in ordinary life and break down some of the stigma surrounding dementia. **This can be evidenced by**: • analysis of activities programme • interviews with staff regarding access to community facilities outside the home • interviews with service users and families.	Excellent Good OK Needs more work

POINTS FOR ACTION	OVERALL PERFORMANCE ON THE SOCIAL ENVIRONMENT

References

Aldridge, D. (2000) *Music Therapy in Dementia Care.* London: Jessica Kingsley Publishers.

Allan, K. and Killick, J. (2000) 'Undiminished possibility: the arts in dementia care.' *Journal of Dementia Care 8*, 3, 16–17.

Alzheimers's Society (2001) *Quality Dementia Care in Care Homes: Person-centred Standards.* London: Alzheimer's Society.

Baker, C.J. and Edwards, P.A. (2002) 'The missing link: benchmarking person-centred care.' *Journal of Dementia Care 10*, 6, 22–3.

Barker, R., Holloway, J., Holtkamp, C.C.M., Larsson, A., Hartman, L.C., Pearce, R., Scherman, B., Johansson, S., Thomas, P.W., Wareing, L.A. and Owens, M. (2003) 'Effects of multi-sensory stimulation for people with dementia.' *Journal of Advanced Nursing 43*, 5, 465–77.

Batson, P. (1998) 'Drama as therapy: bringing memories to life.' *Journal of Dementia Care 6*, 4, 19–21.

Bell, V. and Troxell, D. (1997) *The Best Friends Approach to Alzheimer's Care.* London: Health Professions Press.

Bender, M.P. and Cheston, R. (1997) 'Inhabitants of a lost kingdom: a model for the subjective experiences of dementia.' *Ageing and Society 17*, 513–32.

Bond, J. (2001) 'Sociological perspectives.' In C. Cantley (ed.) *Handbook of Dementia Care.* Buckingham: Open University Press.

Bradford Dementia Group (1997) *Evaluating Dementia Care: The DCM Method*, 7th edition. Bradford: University of Bradford.

Bradford Dementia Group (2005) *DCM 8 User's Manual: The DCM Method*, 8th edition. Bradford: University of Bradford.

Brenner, T. and Brenner, K. (2004) 'Embracing Montessori methods in dementia care.' *Journal of Dementia Care 12*, 3, 24–6.

Brod, M., Stewart, A.L., Sands, L. and Walton, P. (1999) 'Conceptualization and measurement of quality of life in dementia.' *The Gerontologist 38*, 25–35.

Brooker, D. (2004) 'What is person-centred care for people with dementia?' *Reviews in Clinical Gerontology 13*, 3, 215–22.

Brooker, D. (2005) 'Dementia Care Mapping (DCM): a review of the research literature.' *The Gerontologist 45*, 1, 11–18.

Brooker, D. and Surr, C.A. (2005) *Dementia Care Mapping: Principles and Practice.* Bradford: University of Bradford.

Brooker, D. and Surr, C. (2006) 'Dementia Care Mapping (DCM): initial validation of DCM 8 in UK field trials.' *International Journal of Geriatric Psychiatry 21*, 1–8.

Brooker, D., Edwards, P., Benson, S. (eds) (2004) *DCM Experience and Insights into Practice.* London: Hawker Publications.

Brooker, D. and Woolley, R. (in press) 'Enriching opportunities for people living with dementia: the development of a blueprint for a sustainable activity-based model of care.' *Ageing and Mental Health.*

Brooker, D., Woolley, R. and Lee, D. (in press) 'Enriching opportunities for people living with dementia in nursing homes: an evaluation of a multi-level activity-based model of care.' *Ageing and Mental Health.*

Bryden, C. (2005) *Dancing with Dementia: My Story of Living Positively with Dementia.* London: Jessica Kingsley Publishers.

Camp, C.J. and Skrajner, M.J. (2004) 'Resident-Assisted Montessori Programming (RAMP): training persons with dementia to serve as group activity leaders.' *The Gerontologist 44*, 426–31.

Chaudhury, H. (2003) 'Remembering home through art.' *Alzheimer's Care Quarterly 4*, 2, 119–24.

Cheston, R. (1998) 'Psychotherapeutic work with people with dementia: a review of the literature.' *British Journal of Medical Psychology 71*, 3, 211–31.

Clare, L. (2002) 'We'll fight as long as we can: coping with the onset of Alzheimer's disease.' *Aging and Mental Health 6*, 139–48.

Clare, L., Baddeley, A., Moniz-Cook, E. and Woods, R. (2003) 'A quiet revolution.' *The Psychologist 16*, 250–4.

Coaten, R. (2001) 'Exploring reminiscence through dance and movement.' *Journal of Dementia Care 9*, 5, 19–22.

Cohen-Mansfield, J. (2005) 'Nonpharmacological interventions for persons with dementia.' *Alzheimer's Care Quarterly 6*, 2, 129–45.

DASN International www.dasninternational.org. Accessed 24 October 2006.

Department of Health (DH) (2001a) *National Service Framework for Older People.* London: DH.

Department of Health (2001b) *The Essence of Care – Patient Focused Benchmarking for Health Care Practitioners.* London: DH.

Department of Health (2005) *Everybody's Business: Integrated Mental Health Services for Older Adults, A Service Development Guide.* London: Care Services Improvement Partnership (CSIP).

Downs, M. (1997) 'The emergence of the person in dementia research.' *Ageing and Society 17*, 597–607.

Feil, N. (1993) *The Validation Breakthrough.* Cleveland: Health Professions Press.

Finnema, E., Droes, R.-M., Ribbe, M. and van Tilburg, W. (2000) 'The effects of emotion-oriented approaches in the care for persons suffering from dementia: a review of the literature.' *International Journal of Geriatric Psychiatry 15*, 2, 141–61.

Finnema, E., Droes, R.-M., Ettema, T., Ooms, M., Ader, H., Ribbe, M. and van Tilburg, W. (2005) 'The effect of integrated emotion-oriented care versus usual care on elderly persons with dementia in the nursing home and on nursing assistants: a randomized clinical trial.' *International Journal of Geriatric Psychiatry 20*, 4, 330–43.

Garner, P. (2004) 'A SPECAL place to keep.' *Journal of Dementia Care 12*, 3, 11–12.

Gibson, S. (2005) 'A personal experience of successful doll therapy.' *Journal of Dementia Care 13*, 3, 22.

Gigliotti, C.M., Jarrott, S.E. and Yorgason, J. (2004) 'Harvesting health: effects of three types of horticultural therapy activities for persons with dementia.' *Dementia 3*, 2, 161–70.

Goldsmith, M. (1996) *Hearing the Voice of People with Dementia.* London: Jessica Kingsley Publishers.

Gubrium, J. (1989) 'Emotive work and emotive discourse in the Alzheimer's disease experience.' *Current Perspectives on Ageing and the Life Cycle 3,* 243–68.

Hawkins, A.H. (2005) 'Epiphanic knowledge and medicine.' *Cambridge Quarterly of Health Economics 14,* 1, 40–60.

Help the Aged (2006) *My Home Life; Quality of Life in Care Homes.* London: Help the Aged.

Holden, U.P. and Woods, R.T. (1988) *Reality Orientation: Psychological Approaches to the Confused Elderly.* Edinburgh: Churchill Livingstone.

Hughes, J.C. (2001) 'Views of the person with dementia.' *Journal of Medical Ethics 27,* 86–91.

Innes, A. (ed.) (2003) *Dementia Care Mapping: Applications across Cultures.* Baltimore: Health Services Press.

Innes, A., Macpherson, S. and McCabe, L. (2006) *Promoting Person Centred Care at the Front Line.* York: Joseph Rowntree Foundation.

Jarrott, S.E. and Bruno, K. (2003) 'Intergenerational activities involving persons with dementia: an observational assessment.' *American Journal of Alzheimer's Disease and Other Dementias 18,* 1, 31–7.

Keady, J. (1996) 'The experience of dementia: a review of the literature and implications for nursing practice.' *Journal of Clinical Nursing 5,* 275–88.

Killick, J. and Allan, K. (2001) *Communication and the Care of People with Dementia.* Buckingham: Open University Press.

Killick, J. and Allan, K. (2006) 'The Good Sunset Project: Making contact with those close to death.' *Journal of Dementia Care 14,* 1, 22–24.

King's Fund (1986) *Living Well into Old Age: Applying Principles of Good Practice to Services for Elderly People with Severe Mental Disabilities.* London: King's Fund.

Kitwood, T. (1987a) 'Dementia and its pathology: in brain, mind or society?' *Free Associations 8,* 81–93.

Kitwood, T. (1987b) 'Explaining senile dementia: the limits of neuropathological research.' *Free Associations 10,* 117–40.

Kitwood, T. (1988) 'The technical, the personal and the framing of dementia.' *Social Behaviour 3,* 161–80.

Kitwood, T. (1989) 'Brain, mind and dementia: with particular reference to Alzheimer's disease.' *Ageing and Society 9,* 1, 1–15.

Kitwood, T. (1990a) 'The dialectics of dementia: with particular reference to Alzheimer's disease.' *Ageing and Society 10,* 177–96.

Kitwood, T. (1990b) 'Understanding senile dementia: a psychobiographical approach.' *Free Associations 19,* 60–76.

Kitwood, T. (1993a) 'Person and process in dementia.' *International Journal of Geriatric Psychiatry 8,* 7, 541–6.

Kitwood, T. (1993b) 'Towards a theory of dementia care: the interpersonal process.' *Ageing and Society 13,* 1, 51–67.

Kitwood, T. (1993c) 'Discover the person, not the disease.' *Journal of Dementia Care 1,* 1, 16–17.

Kitwood, T. (1995a) 'Positive long-term changes in dementia: some preliminary observations.' *Journal of Mental Health 4*, 2, 133–44.

Kitwood, T. (1995b) 'Building up the mosaic of good practice.' *Journal of Dementia Care 3*, 5, 12–13.

Kitwood, T (1997a) *Dementia Reconsidered: The Person Comes First.* Buckingham: Open University Press.

Kitwood, T. (1997b) 'The uniqueness of persons with dementia.' In M. Marshall (ed.) *State of the Art in Dementia Care.* London: Centre for Policy on Ageing.

Kitwood, T. (1997c) 'The experience of dementia.' *Ageing and Mental Health 1*, 13–22.

Kitwood,T. and Benson, S. (eds) (1995) *The New Culture of Dementia Care.* London: Hawker Publications.

Kitwood, T. and Bredin, K. (1992a) 'Towards a theory of dementia care: personhood and wellbeing.' *Ageing and Society 12*, 269–87.

Kitwood, T. and Bredin, K. (1992b) 'A new approach to the evaluation of dementia care.' *Journal of Advances in Health and Nursing Care 1*, 5, 41–60.

Kitwood, T. and Bredin, K. (1992c) *Person to Person: A Guide to the Care of Those with Failing Mental Powers.* Essex: Gale Centre Publications.

Marshall, M. (2001) 'The challenge of looking after people with dementia.' *British Medical Journal 323*, 410–11.

May, H. and Edwards, P. (in press due 2007) *Person Centred Care Planning: The Milestones Templates.* London: Jessica Kingsley Publishers.

Mezey, M., Boltz, M., Esterton, J. and Mitty, E. (2005) 'Evolving models of geriatric nursing care.' *Geriatric Nursing 26*, 1, 11–15.

Moniz-Cook, E. Stokes, G. and Agar, S. (2003) 'Difficult behavior and dementia in nursing homes: five cases of psychosocial intervention.' *Clinical Psychology and Psychotherapy 10*, 3, 197–208.

Morrisey, M.V. (2006) 'Alzheimer's care for people with and affected by dementia.' *Nursing Times 102*, 15, 29–31.

Morton, I. (1999) *Person-centred Approaches to Dementia Care.* Bicester: Winslow Press Ltd.

Mozley, C.G., Huxley, P., Sutcliffe, C., Bagley, H., Burns, A., Challis, D. and Cordingley, L. (1999) '"Not knowing where I am doesn't mean I don't know what I like": cognitive impairment and quality of life responses in elderly people.' *International Journal of Geriatric Psychiatry 14*, 776–83.

Noelker, L.S. and Ejaz, F.K. (2005) 'Training direct care workers for person-centered care.' *Public Policy and Ageing report 15*, 4, 1–19.

Nolan, M., Davies, S. and Grant, G. (2001) *Working with Older People and Their Families: Key Issues in Policy and Practice.* Buckingham: Open University Press.

Orrell, M., Spector, A., Thorgrimsen, L. and Woods, B. (2005) 'A pilot study examining the effectiveness of Maintenance Cognitive Stimulation Therapy (MCST) for people with dementia.' *International Journal of Geriatric Psychiatry 20*, 5, 446–51.

Orsulic-Jeras, S. Judge, K.S. and Camp, C.J. (2000) 'Montessori-based activities for long-term care residents with advanced dementia: effects on engagement and affecr.' *The Geronotologist 40*, 1, 107–11.

Packer, T. (1996) 'Shining a light on simple, crucial details.' *Journal of Dementia Care 4*, 6, 22–3, Nov/Dec.

Perrin, T. and May, H. (1999) *Well-being in Dementia. An Occupational Approach for Therapists and Carers.* Edinburgh: Churchill Livingstone.

Pioneer Network www.pioneernetwork.net. Accessed 24 October 2006.

Post, S. (1995) *The Moral Challenge of Alzheimer's Disease.* Baltimore: Johns Hopkins University Press.

Pulsford, D., Rushforth, D. and Connor, I. (2000) 'Woodlands therapy: an ethnographic analysis of a small-group therapeutic activity for people with moderate or severe dementia.' *Journal of Advanced Nursing 32*, 3, 650–7.

Rader, J. Doan, J., Schwab, M. (1985) 'How to decrease wandering, a form of agenda behaviour.' *Geriatric Nursing 6*, 4, 196–9.

Rogers, C.R. (1961) *On Becoming a Person.* Boston: Houghton Mifflin.

Sabat, S. (1994) 'Excess disability and malignant social psychology: a case study in Alzheimer's disease.' *Journal of Community and Applied Psychology 4*, 175–66.

Sabat, S. (2001) *The Experience of Alzheimer's Disease: Life through a Tangled Veil.* Oxford: Blackwell.

Sherratt, K., Thornton, A., and Hatton, C. (2004a) 'Music interventions for people with dementia: a review of the literature.' *Aging and Mental Health 8*, 1, 3–12.

Sherratt, K., Thornton, A. and Hatton, C. (2004b) 'Emotional and behavioural responses to music in people with dementia: an observational study.' *Aging and Mental Health 8*, 3, 233–41.

Smallwood, J., Brown, R., Coulter, F., Irvine, E. and Copland, C. (2001) 'Aromatherapy and behaviour disturbances in dementia: a randomized controlled trial.' *International Journal of Geriatric Psychiatry 16*, 10, 1010–13.

Stokes, G. (2000) *Challenging Behaviour in Dementia: A Person-centred Approach.* Bicester: Speechmark Publishing.

Stokes, G. and Goudie, F. (1990) *Working with Dementia.* Bicester: Winslow Press.

Stokes, G. and Goudie, F. (2003) *A Handbook of Dementia Care.* Chichester: John Wiley and Sons.

Thomas, W.H. (1996) *Life Worth Living: How Someone you Love can Still Enjoy Life in a Nursing Home. The Eden Alternative in Action.* Acton, MA: Vanderwyk and Burnam.

Thorgrimsen, L., Spector, A., Wiles, A. and Orrell, M. (2004). *Aromatherapy for Dementia (Cochrane Review).* The Cochrane Library, Issue 2. Oxford: John Wiley and Sons Ltd.

Trilsbach, J. (2002) 'Mary teaches us that caring is a continual learning process.' *Journal of Dementia Care 10*, 3, 22–6.

Verity, J. and Kuhn, D. (in press) *The Art of Good Dementia Care: A Guide for Direct Care Staff in Residential Settings.* New York: Thomas Delmar.

Verkaik, R., Van Weert, J.C.M. and Francke, A.L. (2005) 'The effects of psychosocial methods on depressed, aggressive and apathetic behaviors of people with dementia: a systematic review.' *International Journal of Geriatric Psychiatry 20*, 4, 301–14.

Woods, B., Spector, A., Jones, C., Orrell, M. and Davies, S. (2005) 'Reminiscence therapy for dementia (Cochrane Review).' The Cochrane Database of Systematic Reviews 2005, 2, Art.no.CD 001120.DOI:10.1002/ 14651858.CD001120. (supplement 1), S7–S16.

Subject Index

Author Index

Aldridge, D. 24
Allan, K. 24, 67